Pra
The Heart that

"Barbara's empathy, care and support are apparent on every page."
— *Jackie, Virginia*

"Very interesting, behind the scenes of what nurses do."
— *Carol, Massachusetts*

"This is definitely a book to curl up with."
— *Jessica, RN*

About the Author

"This woman has been in the trenches!"
— *Keli, RN*

"Barbara, Your experience and knowledge is very credible. I trust you on this subject."
— *Deborah, Virginia*

"What I noticed right away as Barbara began to coach me in HeartMath® is that she became calm and centered and totally focused on me. She was not merely teaching me facts she was coaching me in tools to open my heart."
— *Linda, California*

"Barbara is passionate about healing and wholeness which comes across when she lectures. She is warm and engaging and commands the room with her passion and enthusiasm."
— *Linda Gauthier, RN Integrative Healing Arts Practitioner, Reiki Master*

THE HEART THAT ROCKS HEALTH CARE

Nurses - Move from Stress to Success, Empowerment and Influence

Barbara Young, RN

HEARTLIGHT PRESS
FAIR OAKS, CALIFORNIA, USA

ISBN: 978-1-7330269-0-1

Library of Congress Control Number: 2021920324

DISCLAIMER

Neither the author, publisher, editor or cited parties assumes any responsibility for errors, omissions, or contrary interpretations of the subject matter. All included URLs were active and referred to existing websites and information at the time of the first printing. The author put forth all information with the highest integrity, appropriate permissions secured and identities changed. Any other interpretation is unintentional. No medical, legal, psychological, business, financial, religious or other professional advice is contained or implied within this book or related publications, websites, e-mails, presentations, programs, communications, coaching or conversations. In the event you use any of the information in this book, the author and publisher assumes no responsibility.

Brand and product names are trademarks or registered trademarks of their respective owners, including AH SUCCESS Process, Easy as A-B-C technique, and

Editing by Julie Beyers, www.TheWordWrig

Cover Design by David Loofbourrow, Vivo Digital Arts,

Interior Design & Typeset by Vivo Digital Arts, VivoD

Author's Photos by And

Publisher's Note: Third party sales of new and
quality, authority, or access to any in

DEDICATION

For Olive Marie, my precious mom,
who guided me to
make my own milestones in life.
She encouraged me to dream because,
"You have to have a dream
to have a dream come true."

Gosh, I'm a lucky daughter!

☙

CONTENTS

PART TWO
AH SUCCESS 125

PART THREE
Empowerment & Influence 295

FORWARD

I have been blessed in countless ways in this life, but am most grateful for Love. One of the most precious and constant ways that Love has shown up for me is through my forty-year friendship with one of the most enlightening people in my life. She has a lot to share, but is actually very quiet. She does not proclaim her wisdom loudly, but simply whispers the truth to anyone who asks her for clarity. Beneath her serenity lies a fierce warrior for love, justice, inner peace and harmony. I have seen that she is a seeker, far from aimless; she is called from within to attend to the disruptive and disturbing even when others will look away. Time and time again, this inevitably reveals a pearl of insight about how to live better and healthier in our times.

I met Barbara Young when I was an eighteen-year-old Kentucky transplant to Orlando. We were getting ready to enter the nursing program at the University of Central Florida. Even though Barbara was a year younger, I knew right away that she was mature beyond her years. We shared a past of difficult childhoods that cultivated in both of us a strong dependence on self and immediately bonded as truth seekers, trying to make sense of a confusing world and land on our feet somewhere inside adulthood. I didn't know it at the time, but Barbara would go on to play an invaluable role in my life. I am forever grateful to know and love her.

Barbara entered nursing full of optimism and insatiable curiosity. I found the education logical and methodical, and while she got that too, she always asked questions bigger than the curricula. Continuing education classes were not only the way to keep her RN license current through the years, but a way of satisfying her endless desire to learn. She reached beyond the defined job of conventional nursing practice to embrace complimentary skills, such as massage therapy and meditation. From these she learned fundamentals of healing and health which resonated with the roots of nursing. I knew she had found her niche when she wove holistic principles into her hospital-based critical and emergent nursing care, that was later rewarded with recognition from the American Holistic Nurses Association as a Board Certified Holistic Nurse, by review of a portfolio of her life's work.

Though I began my clinical career in high-risk labor and delivery within a hospital, within five years I joined a midsize publicly-traded company using remote monitoring technology that allowed high-risk pregnant women to stay at home safely versus spend weeks or months in a hospital room. Telemedicine quickly became a passion for me, as did leadership. I also found that I had a knack for "selling" when I believed in something and so I crossed over from a purely clinical role to one in combination with the business side of healthcare. I quickly learned how to run a company 'by the numbers' from my boss, the CEO, who came from a background in finance.

As an aspiring executive, I was scared of what I didn't know. I had the confidence and ability to think my way through most situations, but nothing substituted for my lack of experience. My response was to become bigger, more intimidating, and more demanding. It was little wonder that I was not liked by those who reported to me, even as they admired my work.

In my darkest times of reckoning, it was Barbara who was there to hold a loving, safe space for me to finally turn toward the mirror. She offered her love and wisdom from her experience about peace, perspective, self-love and self-care throughout, even when I resisted.

I joked about dancing with the dark side, but Barbara saw a beauty in the dance steps, crossing back and forth amongst clinical knowledge, business objectives and financial results. I had a chance as a nurse to bring a nursing perspective to the business side of medicine.

Facing my authentic self, applying the knowledge I gained from Barbara, had a profound impact on the path I chose to walk from that point forward. Simply put, as Love became the foundation of my life, the newfound gentle, unassuming, unconditional embrace of humanity offered me the opportunity to inspire and motivate those who worked with me simply by focusing on their success instead of my own. As my love for myself and others grew, so did my success in business.

I watched the path of Barbara's career traverse the diversity of culture, and medical and nursing practice in critical care hospital units of small towns, big cities and on remote islands, as a traveling nurse. I witnessed her blossom into a successful, independent nurse-clinician respected by physicians and admired by co-workers. I realized her career had become her vocation. I admired her devotion to holistic nursing and a health-promoting lifestyle.

During my career, Barbara marveled at my corporate ladder climb and admired my ability to mentally walk the razor's edge of technological innovation and sound clinical practice as a business manager. In my work I felt powerless to change disparities in healthcare that often contributed to frustration and stress for nurses. But Barbara knew that she and her patients had the innate capacity for well-being and she hoped, someday, the medical healthcare model would embrace an approach to maintain health from birth to death. Her yearning for the right environment to support holistic nursing practice and health brought some agonizing days and sleepless nights as the current disease-focused system failed to fulfill her definition of health care time after time.

As technology advanced, the associated faster pace pushed her, and like many clinicians, her way of practice was challenged to prioritize the clock over patients. Over those years, we had many conversations after yet another frustrating shift, with her nurse's heart breaking from being dismissed and misunderstood by the very system she chose for her life's work. She became exhausted instead of energized, frustrated instead of fulfilled, and concerned about her peers who felt the same way she did.

Thankfully, my friend – often humming along the way – walks to her own (heart) beat, no matter the forces trying to control her stride. She has always been intuitive, imaginative, creative and resilient. While feeling grateful for her innate ability to see the future before the rest of us, she would inevitably feel somewhat defeated when it seemed that no one understood. Yet within a few years, her vision materialized or an idea was put into practice in several healthcare settings.

Over the years, I learned to take careful mental note of her ideas because I knew I would see them come to fruition in time. For example, Barbara's quest for a "whole" nursing practice began before I had ever even heard of the concept and before holistic nursing was a specialty in nursing. She, like other early lamp-bearers, sought to actively integrate these concepts into nurses' conventional role. She also sensed the imminent ground swell of job-related stress nurses would suffer.

Simply stated, Barbara has never let what IS interfere with her vision of what COULD BE.

Barbara helped me navigate many painful events in my life as her knowledge of spirituality and personal evolution grew over time. She introduced me to the writings of wisdom keepers and spiritual teachers, helping me to understand that we are more than what we seem on the outside and that the secrets of happiness lie within us, if we'll only believe and look for them. Our conversations overflow with the deepest understanding of truth, and have illuminated my path for 40 years during times of happiness and peace, as well as those of betrayal and pain.

I climbed the corporate ladder in the healthcare industry with footholds stabilized by the wisdom we culminated together, including decision making, management style, relationship building, employee support, team-building, and productivity, as well as patient care program development and self-care for myself and employees.

We continue to find it interesting that we took such different paths with the same nursing education. Though the scenes of our lives and careers looked so different, the celebrations and trials revealed lessons so similar for each of us that we sometimes felt like one person living two lives.

From the first days of our meeting in Florida all those years ago, Barbara has dreamed out loud of being an author. She kept ideas on scraps of paper and notes in the margins of books she read alluding to what she might write about someday. She even kept a list of potential titles.

However, until she hung up her scrubs in retirement, her life had no room for writing despite her desire. Success called in the form of a painfully difficult good-bye to a career that no longer served her growth, even as Barbara was, at times, uncertain of exactly what steps to take next. She followed her dream, took a writing course that set deadlines upon her, and finally began to write. Her inner voice started to sing and the results spilled out on the following pages.

Amazed, as I first read her words, it reinforced for me that there is wisdom in patience and faith, and truly a time for everything under Heaven. When I read from her initial manuscript to my mother, a second mother to Barbara, my mother asked, "How did she write this?" I answered, "She was born to write this."

So I ask on behalf of your beautiful, nursing soul: please open your truth-and-health-seeking-heart and hum along with Barbara on your journey.

— Susan B. Riley
Healthcare Executive
Sedona, Arizona

PREFACE

"Nurses are the conduit of care that allows any profession, hospital, business, organization or technology to touch people."

— Barbara Young, RN
   publisher, "Nurses Moving Forward-
   Innovation with Heart" (2014)

You know the feeling, that tugging in your inner core that won't let go. Something isn't right, is it? Where is that feeling for you? The gut is a common part of one's body that communicates in this way. Is it telling you something isn't adding up, you need to be cautious, true to yourself… or perhaps that you are stressed-out? Your gut may have even recruited more influential partners to activate your inner call light, resulting in neck or back pain, or even raising your blood pressure. Your body will do whatever it takes to get your attention, even create *dis-ease*.

Your body will make you aware that it is unhappy. Awareness is often the first step on a path to success. It is likely one reason you are reading this book. What are you seeking? It could be answers, solutions, options, camaraderie, validation, healing or work-life balance. Even if you do not know exactly what you are seeking, with the help of this book you are well on your way to finding it.

You, my colleague, are why I wrote this book and created the AH SUCCESS Process. I have been looking forward to collaborating with you about our jobs, stress and health. What I wrote in these pages draws from my personal and professional experience, synthesized from the knowledge and wisdom of multiple disciplines, and the works of leading-edge researchers and teachers. Together, we will go through the steps so you can transform your stress into success.

In my professional career I have been *walking* with people toward their success for many years. Since the early 1980s, through teaching, consulting and coaching about well-being, stress, self-empowerment, and dream realization, I have witnessed honesty, courage and determination in people moving toward their vision of health and well-being. I have cared for people using advanced technology in critical, cardiac and emergent care, and amidst profound simplicity on an island without a hospital. As a nurse, my jobs have each been a blessing. They gave me access to a venue for my work and people who needed nursing care. Isn't that what called you into nursing… the desire to help people?

Whether I coach for well-being or care for people under medical treatment, I feel called to be present with and advocate for the spirit of that person, as do you. While you stand strong for others when they are weak, ailing or vulnerable, who does so for you? I hear the whimpers of your dampened spirit. The burdens related to your job environment have taken a toll on your well-being.

The job of a nurse has always been challenging, but for today's nurse it has become is more complex, multifaceted, demanding, even dangerous. You continue to become more educated and experienced, along with accepting more responsibility and liability. People are getting sicker and the healthcare system is busier. The impacts of technology are challenging. Deeper than all this, something fundamental in the terrain of your job has changed. You sense it. You feel its effects. But what is it? What can or should you do?

Perhaps we can look to the past for clues. Do you recall the "Job Switching" episode in Season 2 of *I Love Lucy* where Lucy and Ethel get a job at a chocolate factory? Are you already laughing? If you do not recall this show, please search for it online and watch it. If you remember it, consider watching it again and enjoy a hearty laugh; it is de-stressing.

If you have not seen it or cannot look it up, I will brief you. Lucy and Ethel have just started at a job where their task is wrapping a paper around each piece of candy that goes by on a conveyor belt. They are anxious with anticipation, but once the belt moves, they get into a flow. Just as they comment to each other that this is something they can handle and they seem to enjoy it, guess what happens? The belt picks up speed, so they speed up. It increases more and they change their method to keep up. Pace continues to increase and they are both showing distress, but they have to get the job done.

They get creative on ways to make it look like everything is working and ensure that no unwrapped candies are getting past them. Then the boss comes around and there's a scramble. What the boss sees is that everything is operational and no candies are going unwrapped – they are doing a good job. Based upon this short-sighted conclusion, the boss gives the command to speed up the conveyor belt even more. It is still only Lucy and Ethel working the line. Can you relate?

It may not be easy to realize that the job they hired you for is, by description, one that your employer ideals and certain laws define. Accepting the job and its description did not make you a nurse. They hired you because you are a nurse, trained to do the tasks of the job. Your call to nurse was likely in your heart, even before you went to nursing school to get the training to work as one. You hoped the career you chose would validate your giving nature and let you do what you felt destined to do.

What you seek is a manager who is authentic and encourages the best of you, a transformational leader who builds a healthy work environment for nurses and healing. Your need for hydration, nutrition, elimination and rest while on-the-job is just as valid as the need for an environment free of hostility with open communication and implementation of your ideas, according to Rose E. Sherman, EdD, RN, FAAN, in her *Emerging Leaders* article, "What Do Nurses Want from Their Leaders?".[1]

It's true administration pressures managers, but you need your manager to advocate for you and what you need to get your job done. If for no other reason, when you get your job done, it makes her look like she has done a good job. Carrots and sticks to motivate nurses and cute thank-you gifts like pens or mugs can be successful to a point. But what you really want are breaks, restful sleep, authority, respect and work-life balance.

Leadership expert John Maxwell, in his book *The 21 Irrefutable Laws of Leadership,* states, "The proof of leadership is found in followers."[2] So if you and your co-workers are making mistakes, burning out, becoming ill, frustrated or complaining, it is reasonable to consider the workplace environment and its leadership as contributing to these issues. The first paradox is that you have more power than you think. You can make your own choices and you also influence others as a role model. The second is that you are a leader. Turn around and look into your life starting with your job, family and social circle. Look at all who look to you – who you care for, guide and encourage. Be willing to accept that credit. Be open to grow into the person who the author of *Dare to Lead: Brave Work, Tough Conversations, Whole Hearts*, Brené Brown, calls a "daring leader".[3]

Everything seems backwards, inside out or upside down. Healthcare needs to learn from the causes of illness and teach people how to perpetuate health as a way of living. Likewise, a manager's priority needs to be the well-being of her staff nurses so they can care for the patients. It seems those in administration ought to ask you what you need to do your job, which would lead to more satisfaction for you and your patients. In this way management can fulfill their goals for patient care, nurse retention and their bottom line. They need you. No matter how much tangible technology they purchase, it cannot replace you at the bedside. If that were possible, what would that mean for those who need safe, monitored nurse-administered medical treatments and nursing care?

You deliver their medical treatments safely and timely, with compassion and a smile, no matter how many obstacles you have to overcome to do so. Your calling is to be at the patient's side through their uncertainty and vulnerability. Patients need your presence, touch, and eyes of depth, warmth and honesty. They need to feel understood and to know you will see them through their ordeal. You are deeply valuable as their advocate and overseer of their safe passage through their medical treatments. Gallup Poll surveys have shown that nurses are the most trusted professional and have been every year since 1999, except for the year of the firefighter in 2001. Voted on by the people they serve, nurses maintain this high honor with even higher scores each year, for honesty and ethical standards. Despite this achievement, many of your sister and brother colleagues join in chorus with your inner chant. They feel under-appreciated and stressed on the job. When the 2014 Nurses

Stress Survey, by The Vickie Milazzo Institute, revealed its findings, several sources reported the results as "alarming". According to the survey, the effects of feeling "overworked without relief in sight" with "people telling you how to do your job… who have lost sight of patient care" while having "responsibility but no authority" where there is "corporate chaos, greed and mismanagement" and "working in a system that is broken" are showing up as stress and illness for you and your colleagues.

Why don't *they* move out of the way and let you do what you need to do? What if *they* did? What if the tumultuous arena of mainstream medical healthcare opened up to you and you could command how it proceeds? What would you want? What is the value you bring as a nurse to your job, medicine and health? How would you address pressing issues like the overall declining health of people and health of nurses, and the increasing patient volume and acuity? What if now was the time that, as a nurse, *they* would listen to you? These are important questions to ponder and possibilities to entertain.

Ideally, you will find answers to these and other self inquires as you read this book and take part in the AH SUCCESS Process. Feeling powerless does not contribute to good health outcomes for you. Being without the power to change, influence and direct patient care does not contribute to good health outcomes for your patients. What is the power that you need?

Your angst is telling you something. There is urgency because you are beyond being uncomfortable. While nurses have always risked a broken heart through loss of people in their care, their jobs evolved to compete with construction work for risk of injury, and now research links stress to the six leading causes of death – and your instincts tell you that your situation is not sustainable.

Marianne Williamson has been a long-time inspirational mentor for me. She reveals the depth of why I wrote this book. In her poem "Our Deepest Fear" she states, "Our deepest fear is that we are powerful beyond measure." She challenges, "Who are you *not* to be?" (emphasis mine) because, "…playing small does not serve the world." Williamson affirms that "…as we let our light shine… As we're liberated from our own fear, our presence automatically liberates others."[4]

Pause and breathe that message in. As you shine, you give others permission to shine. There is no competition; all are meant to shine. Do you feel a calling or nudge to go beyond mere survival to thrive as your amazing self – personally, vocationally, professionally, and in health? This is about fully being an emissary for health for yourself and those around you.

You are seeking and readying yourself to take action on your discoveries. In this book I will walk with you toward your empowerment, from stress to success. When you get the answers to your stress, you will inevitably lead those you love and care for in discovering theirs.

Heart to heart,

Barbara

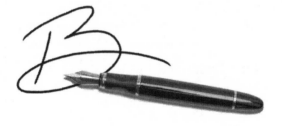

INTRODUCTION

The Heart that Rocks Health Care is an empowerment book for nurses to transform their stress into success, because, as The HeartMath Institute has confirmed, "A change in heart changes everything." It is deeply concerning, that the burden and fatigue from stress is causing heart-felt suffering for nurses. They need tools of empowerment to cultivate a change of heart toward health for themselves and health care.

Consider this book an explorative discussion, including yourself as an integral part of the dialog, which will go on between us and within your head, heart, body and soul. Hopefully, the topics will also become a dialog between you and your colleagues.

Your heart will be your best guide as you read this book because it naturally makes connections where the brain may judge and disconnect. Your heart knows your true nature which tends toward healing.

Allow yourself to experience this book with an open mind and heart. As you read, allow yourself to dwell in possibility. This can be a cozy journey through this book for you and your heart, even when it challenges your mind to stretch. I weave information throughout this book in such a manner that you can hopefully experience it more than rationalize it. This leads to redundancy of some concepts to build understanding, reinforce progress, and show continuity. While explaining or describing things, when the usual or common words are inadequate I make up my own. Those and other words that need emphasis or are uncommon will be in *italics*, and if needed, will have an endnote with additional information.

I wrote from my own perspective, as if speaking to a seasoned staff nurse, and use the feminine pronouns to keep it simple, consistent and personal. I did this without the intent to exclude or specifically include.

Anyone who identifies with or is curious about the roles and topics explored will benefit from the content in this book. We are all beings of love and light. Limited perceptions, labels, and pronouns make us seem separate, different and fragmented. In this writing, I intend to honor both uniqueness and universality despite grammatical formalities.

This is an integrative journey you are on; the information is valuable. To avoid overload, get the lesson and move forward. You need to metabolize your stress, just as your body transforms food into energy and vitality while eliminating anything unnecessary. Have fresh water available to drink periodically while reading to facilitate this, and to refresh your mind.

Your heart will be your best guide as you read and experience this book because it naturally makes connections where the brain may judge and disconnect. Your heart knows your true nature which naturally tends toward healing.

In my career as a cardiac care nurse, my colleagues and I observed denial to be 'an early sign of a heart attack' when it occurred with chest pressure, dismissed as indigestion. Do not underestimate any potential indications of a need for professional care. The information presented is for self-care, health promotion and empowerment that can become your lifestyle or complement other professional care. **If you experience chest pain, gastrointestinal pain, concerning headaches, sleep and mood issues, fatigue, pain, and any number of other symptoms, do not use this information as or to replace medical diagnosis, advice or treatment, nor to replace any other professional care.** Hopefully you are answering your inner call light timely, but do not ignore that often endocrine, micronutrient, cellular, even mitochondrial depletion from stress is so severe that supplementation and medical rescue is necessary.

This book is written in three sections:

Part One is an exploratory and informational conversation about stress and its determinants including the environment you work in. This will serve as validation and preparation for you to discover the power you have inside to answer your inner call light.

Part Two is a comprehensive, conceptual and experiential journey, as I lead you through the nine steps of the AH SUCCESS Process which are based upon fundamental principles of manifestation applied to moving from stress to success. I recommend you process the information through experience, be the proof, and keep learning.

Part Three reveals your empowerment and influence which lay beyond the cauldron of stress and how there is no time like now to move forward into health and success.

Throughout this book, you will find paragraphs that start with a heart symbol. These heart activities, like the one below, are within the text to facilitate interaction or reflection as part of the experience of reading this book. In the heart paragraphs you will find questions, activities, and information for consideration, exploration, experience, and to take to heart. I hope that you will find them engaging and be compelled to record your answers and related thoughts, questions, ideas, dreams and self-expressions.

For this, I recommend you have a journal. It can be as practical as a pad of paper or bound journal book, as savvy as an app, or as personal as a decorated book of handmade paper. The important thing is that your journal is useful and accessible as you read this book. Something may move you to write in your journal spontaneously, and I encourage you to follow your heart on this. The information in the journal is for you alone unless you share it by choice. Some parts you may refer to again, but it is also okay to release into the pages and not look at it again.

As a warm-up for moving from stress to success, let's start by lightening your load. At the top of a page in your journal, write "My Stress" as the heading. If you can ID it, you can be free of it, so list what stresses you.

I mean for this to be a stress dump, so use as many pages as you need – get them off your heart and out of your mind for now. You will refer back to this list during other heart activities. It is okay if you want to leave an open page or two for anything that you may wish to add later. Make your list, then sigh as you say, "AH," ease your shoulders and leave your stress on the pages of your journal.

It takes the power of your will – your power of self-determination – as 'the heart that rocks health care' to carve out time to counterbalance the treadmill of your life. Your time with this book is an accomplishment of just that, as an investment in yourself – your most valuable asset. It takes courage to allow yourself to retreat, which is often necessary to advance. As you turn each page, you take a step forward.

**Look for the ⓘ symbol which indicates
supporting materials are available.**

**You will find it convenient to
download them now at:**

https://BYoungBooks.com/support-heart

PART ONE

STRESS: EPIDEMIC OR NEW WAY OF LIFE?

S tress has been undermining people's health for decades. Science is defining how stress leads to early infirmity and even death. Now it is coming to light that stress is dramatically attacking the ones needed to take care of people when they get sick.

Part One explores the many ways stress is claiming the health and well-being of the most hardy of people – nurses.

As a nurse, you are familiar with the challenges of stress – it's accepted as part of your job. Though when undefined, unacknowledged or un-managed, stress can slowly destroy you personally and professionally. But your inner call light is frantically flashing and who is responding?

Take the time to discover how and why you are burning out. Identify how stress intermingles in the environment of the caring business you work in and explore opportunities to *de-stress*.

Because there is no quick fix or magic pill, it is critical that you examine the intricacies of the problem. The chapters in Part One will help you survey the environment of your stress and validate your experience. This will prepare you to discover the power you have inside to answer your inner call light.

Now you begin your journey toward relief and success.

CHAPTER 1

STRESS IS A SYMPTOM

You feel stressed and you are not alone. Meet Lee Ann and peek into her life. Does this resemble your workday mornings?

The alarm clock sounds loud on this dark winter morning. Lee Ann tries to get up but her arm won't even move to press snooze. She feels far away from the reality of the workday that lies ahead – warm and comfy in a cocoon of blankets. It feels protective from the increasing acuities at work and shifts without a break. Today will be her fifth shift in a row. But at this moment, the overtime pay is no incentive to get out of bed.

What was I thinking when I agreed to do this extra shift? I care for my colleagues and I don't want them to work short-staffed. They'd rather work short before having the manager step in if I'm not there. What about my patients?

Sighing, her mind wanders to all the things left undone last night.

…dishes, laundry, bedtime reading with the children…

She was so tired she crashed on the couch after dinner. Smiling, she feels thankful for her husband who got both her and their children to bed.

If only I had the energy to be more attentive to my family… but I'm drained after my shift. It seems like every time there is a tournament or performance for the kids or a family gathering, I have to be at work. My children are growing up so fast. I've missed a lot of holiday dinners because I 'had to work.' Murphy's Law? Bad luck?

Karma? Or is there favoritism in the shift scheduling?

As she drifts between wakefulness and sleep, she watches herself in a dream having to leave her pajama-clad family to go into work on a Sunday morning. Rising to the daily work challenges, she systematically switches into her determined-nurse mode.

While at work, I often feel my life is going on without me, as if I am in an alternate life, she observes.

Her gut clenches in confirmation of what she realizes.

The levity in my job is gone. Everyone is too busy and under too much pressure...

Hmm, my headache hasn't started yet. How did I get so tired? Maybe it's because every day there seems to be a new process and practice change on the job. Or it could be technology overload. It seems to have intercepted and diluted what used to be person-to-person relationships, communication and planning related to patient care. And the acuity keeps increasing along with the pace it demands... Just like the other day when the Chief Nursing Officer (CNO) appeared in my patient's room, trying to hasten the suddenly decided discharge because another patient was already waiting in the hall for the room. Maybe after twenty years, my job has caught up with me.

She searches for a feeling of being appreciated.

Oh my, I am totally stressed-out! Am I headed for the same fate as my patients with ulcers, hypertension and chronic disease?

Nuzzling her face deeper into her pillow, Lee Ann dozes as she silently declares,

Sleep is my new favorite thing.

Her husband awakens her.

Okay, I can do this.

She summons her will and gets up for work.

Can you relate to Lee Ann's experience? It doesn't seem like much has improved since 1983, when *Time* magazine published an article calling stress "the epidemic of the eighties" with job stress as the leading cause for adults.[1,2] It may not surprise you that by the mid twenty-teens, the World Health Organization claimed stress to be the "health epidemic of the 21st century."[3]

But how can this be? Who's taking care of peoples' health?

Prevailing Western healthcare practice is to define what is wrong with Lee Ann and give her a diagnosis which dictates the interventions used to treat her. If stress is Lee Ann's diagnosis, how might she treat it on her own? Take a day off or take a hot bath, go for a run, take a vacation or eat a box of chocolates? How well do those things work for you? Do they cure your stress?

How would your doctor treat your stress? It would likely depend upon what your symptoms are. Lee Ann, for example, may get a prescription for pain, another for anxiety, maybe one for mood elevation... perhaps a referral for psychological consultation. How do you think these would work for her? Will it cure her stress? Will her stress ever get resolved? Treated medically with pills and talk therapy, some symptoms may subside, but will the treatments address the actual issues that caused her stress? Probably not. Her stress may continue and become chronic. Then she might get diagnosed with depression, chronic fatigue and ulcers. The current treatment model labels things, and labels tend to stick. Labels would transform Lee Ann from experiencing symptoms related to stress, into being a stressed person. Identification in this way is dis-empowering due to lack of attention to the causes.

A Different Perspective

Consider Lee Ann's stress as a symptom rather than a diagnosis. That would allow her to uncover multiple possible causes. What if the causes were addressed directly? Could the stress and its signs diminish using minimal, short-term or no medications at all? Since both stress and side effects from medications threaten health, could it be prudent to minimize both? Only treatments that address the correct cause will have lasting benefit beyond symptom suppression. In the biology-based systems approach of functional medicine, the focus is on identifying and addressing the root cause of disease.[4]

In this book, I present a holistic and person-focused approach, which is functional rather than medically based, to help you identify your stressors, symptoms and root causes. Do not delay or omit any medical or other professional care needed, however. If your stress is a symptom with deeper causes, learning to listen to it may help you find resolution.

I learned about the functional perspective much later in my nursing career, though it resonated more with the theory-based model of nursing practice taught in my bachelor degree program. Remember those nursing diagnoses which address functional health patterns and basic human needs in terms of alteration, deficiency, effectiveness, impairment or distress?

Heart disease was on the rise when I was a new-grad cardiac care nurse with the lofty dream of helping to heal people's hearts. The suggested correlation of the Type A personality with coronary heart disease fascinated me.[5] With the help of my minor in psychology, I twirled this connection around in my head until I made sense of it. I mused that if they linked certain behaviors to such a lethal disease, why was medicine not teaching people how to cope and make healthier choices to prevent illness? Learning about diet and lifestyle *after* a heart attack seemed backward to me. This realization helped focus my career on the unique role of a nurse – to model and educate on the cultivation of health and the prevention of illness.

(♡) What symptoms of stress are you experiencing? Perhaps you have palpitations, tension in your shoulders, become talkative, or feel impatient. Make a list in your journal, include those physical, emotional, subjective and objective.

Have you heard the adage, "Don't shoot the messenger"? It is a common reaction to lash out or even mount a full-blown attack when given information or feedback that clashes with what you consider acceptable and desirable. That said, I will present things that will challenge your beliefs, education, paradigms and even motivation. Much of the information will seem novel. However, modern scientists are confirming what some cultures have known and practiced for thousands of years and understanding is rapidly expanding. They are developing a new language for the evolving paradigm. Many clients have found the information and skills I will share with you transformational when applied in their life, job, health and relationships. Please don't shoot down the concept too quickly. You may also feel that you *know* this stuff already. You do not need another thing on your to-do list or to feel guilty about not doing. But *something is wrong*, right? Stress can undermine even the most conscientious people and nurses. I am sensitive to this and respect your act of courage to seek answers.

Though many have gone before you, the journey from stress to success can be as unique as the individual walking the path. Because true knowledge lies beyond what is taught or common, it takes effort to explore, understand and apply. Even Plato's theory of knowledge agrees it involves a lot of introspection. The knowledge you gain from self-awareness and *self-regulation* will illuminate and energize your path toward regaining your vitality and realizing your empowerment.[6] Your immune and nervous systems can determine in an instant if something is a threat. This quick determination is a lifesaving measure, made without the consent of your reasoning brain. For survival, this leads to a discharge of the sympathetic nervous system, a process which works great to mount a fight in a bacterial or viral invasion of the body or to alarm us and mobilize the resources needed to flee from a predator. But it is less effective and can be detrimental in the bigger picture of health if it is repeatedly, frequently and unnecessarily activated as it is with chronic stress.

Another way to activate the sympathetic nervous system is by your thoughts and reactions. This process is very sensitive, and it only takes the *perception* of a threat – whether accurate – to activate it. The perception can be unique to you or common and easily validated, as in many modern social situations and business cultures. Realizing an overlooked mortgage payment when a late notice arrives in the mail, seeing a police car suddenly appear in the rear-view mirror or getting called into the manager's office are examples of common situations that may elicit a sympathetic nervous system response. Thoughts in the brain drive this life-protective physiology, even if only as a coping mechanism to get through the challenges of an average day.

No one wants to have stress or symptoms, but both can point toward a path of healing and regaining health. Perhaps you listed a headache as a symptom of stress while at work. If you take a medication to stop the headache and it is successful, you continue working. You trust the medicine, believing relief is coming, and soon it probably does. It is important to do what is necessary to continue to work. But what caused the headache? Was there a message in the headache? Could you gain information that would make it possible to prevent a reoccurrence? Symptoms can be messengers of stress, so don't shoot the messenger. Rather, receive the message that could address the less obvious cause that might lie in the environment.

Environment is Key

Environments can be external, internal, social, philosophical, political, economic, mental, emotional, physical, even spiritual. They can be man-made or natural, involve temperature, altitude and moisture, and they can be healthy or toxic. Causes of stress and illness often lie within the environments influencing a person. This may be conceptually different from what you are accustomed to in the medical knowledge of your job. However, it is foundational to the model of functional medicine.

From a functional medicine perspective, symptoms may be as distant, metaphorically, from their root cause, as the leaves of a tree are distant to the roots and soil' environment. Symptoms are indicators of deeper issues which can be environmental, preceding genetics or infection. If the leaves of a fruit tree are unhealthy – curling, bumpy and shaped irregularly – the common 'medical-type' approach would be to treat the symptoms directly as a disease. Aiming chemicals, radiation and blades at the symptoms, rather than the cause, may lead to a reoccurrence. Or worse, there could be loss of other functions such as providing shade and fruit. Where is the real problem? How can it be found and addressed? If the interventions aimed at the leaves and branches fail, perhaps it's in the roots which sprouted from the original seed that contained its DNA. But if it is in the DNA, how was the tree able to yield delicious, healthy fruit and leaves for many years before the symptoms appeared? What went wrong? Perhaps the cause is in the environment? Does the soil contain the proper nutrients? Is it moist with balanced drainage? Could it be poor air quality, the change in growing seasons, a lack of sun or pruning and tending that has contributed to its weakening? These environmental elements can debilitate the tree by causing imbalances which lead to disease. This is where functional medicine aims to assess and intervene.

Nature, including our bodies, tends toward health. If the environment cannot support healthy growth or otherwise blocks, inhibits or taxes a natural system, it may influence altered-genetic expression, malnutrition, deficiencies, malignancies, malformation, even degradation toward death. Through its amazing propensity to survive and ability to adapt to stress, the tree, in the example above, can adapt to a point of weakness and breakdown, becoming an unwilling host to an infection. Treating the invading organism is a quick intervention, but it does not address the deeper, organic causes that facilitated the development of the conditions that allowed the invader to thrive. If the cause of the condition still exists, the symptoms may only be in remission and the bumpy leaves may reappear. This shows how the environment has a key role in stress and health. The outward, attention-getting bumpy leaf symptoms are the messengers and the result of enduring a threatened homeostasis (environment) which is stressful and needs to be resolved. By shooting the messenger (symptoms), you can lose the clues to the cause.

(♋) Choose a work-stress related symptom from your list to explore for potential messages. Consider your symptom, perhaps a headache or a manager who is hostile.

When you put your attention on the situation or symptom, what happens? Notice any immediate and initial impressions and reactions. Ask yourself exploratory and soft questions, which are ones with no right or wrong answer. *Why this [symptom or situation]? How does this relate to my stress, my success?* Notice what comes up for you.

Responses should arise rather than come from logistics. The simplest and most subtle sensations, including feeling resistance around this exploration, can be a message. How to interpret these messages will come from within you.

Whatever gets your attention increases. With symptoms, it is not uncommon for them to worsen or for more to appear, like more attention given to a child in a tantrum child can exacerbate their behavior. Addressing the root cause does not have to be a direct assault. Sometimes acknowledging it will disarm it.

The result is an absence of symptoms and rebalancing of causative factors. Once resolved, there is better potential to prevent any more symptoms to develop. It is not wrong to address the symptoms, but likely limiting to only do so.

The basis of the predominant model for problem solving, including in healthcare, is Louis Pasteur's theory – to find and target the germ causing the problem The resulting attempts to resolve a problem and provide treatments are episodic and aimed at the proverbial germ or the symptoms. Hence the symptom in any circumstance, whether an employee in a workplace situation or a fever, becomes the focus of all the interventions usually aimed at removing it. This model can be potentially dismissive by not considering that the germ itself may be a symptom of an underlying causal issue.

In recent years there has been a *shift* in medical healthcare toward looking *upstream* from the symptoms for a precursory cause of modern day chronic illnesses, especially when there is no tangible germ and only symptoms. Emphasis is being placed upon genetics, but not so far as considering lifestyle, environment and stress. Ideally, these perspectives of allopathic and functional medicine would complement one another to achieve better outcomes, better toleration of treatment, less reoccurrence and reduced healthcare costs.

It was no doubt unexpected when Louis Pasteur ultimately admitted, "The microbe (germ) is nothing. The terrain (milieu)is everything."[7,8] This is a significant revelation from one who devoted his life to preventing disease by stalking germs, and who's renowned for his discoveries leading to pasteurization and vaccination, Environment is "the aggregate of surrounding things, conditions, or influences; surroundings; milieu."[9] This is why we will look in detail at environmental contributions to your stress.

Genes do their thing in an environment which is life- and health-sustaining or -depleting, hence conducive or not for *dis-ease*. So, what causes the symptoms? The germ or the environment that provided for the growth of the germ? The gene or the environment that influenced the gene-expression? These questions are strikingly similar to the those of the behavioral psychology debate of nature vs. nurture involving the role of environment in personality and human behavior development.[10]

A 2018 documentary by Tim Wardle, *Three Identical Strangers*, reveals the heartwarming reunion story of triplets separated at birth in one such double-blind study. However, it also reveals the tragic answer to the research question about the influence of socioeconomic environment on the development of genetically identical siblings.

Pretend an itchy, bumpy rash appears on your forearm. What are your thoughts about it? Are they aimed at the symptoms or a potential cause? How would you take care of it? If you use a cream to stop the itching, what might it mean if the itching subsides but the bumps persist? Do you see the rash as a symptom or just the itching? Could the bumps also be a symptom? Could your body be detoxifying through its largest excretory organ, your skin? Could it be your immune system is acting appropriately by attempting to alert you? An anti-inflammatory cream or pill may successfully treat the symptoms, but what about the cause? Was there an irritant in your laundry soap, or something inflammatory to your body in some food that you ate? Have you had a similar situation? Use your journal to record any insights.

Ultimately, anything found in the environment, internal or external, could be a cause which would require targeted intervention. If the body is acting appropriately in response to it, masking the annoying symptoms eliminates the means of communicating there is a problem. This can also apply to your experiences of stress. As you resolve the cause, symptom resolution should follow.

Perhaps this knowledge compels you to be more curious about your environment, stress and health. Why are environments of strain, tension and conflict so prevalent? Understanding the concept of environment is achieved by considering many levels of perspective. Each type of environment has a field of influence and effect. They overlap, interplay, counterbalance, resonate and may clash with one another resulting in different outcomes. Let's look at different environments and explore their effects on health. As we do, consider them for yourself and continue to explore your responses and any effects.

CHAPTER 2

MODERN MEDICAL HEALTHCARE ENVIRONMENT

During the 1980s, beepers and fax machines were becoming popular in the business world, including medicine. Characteristically, cardiac patients (generally all males at the time) would worry about checking messages on their beepers within minutes after coming to the unit from a heart catheterization. Despite having just endured a heart attack they could not put themselves first for even a moment. It seemed like they somehow developed a trigger or fetish for these gadgets. Their need for tending to the gadgets kept them on sympathetic alert.[1] They checked them like a day trader checks the stock market.

Who knew this would escalate to the magnitude of device tending and electromagnetic exposure of today? In recent years, research proves that the jingles and beeps are Pavlovian,[2] providing release of both pleasure and stress hormones from the users' brains. This phenomenon has adverse affects on the attention spans and behaviors of children, integrity in relationships and quality of sleep. It has progressed to the point of intentional device-free zones and unplugged vacations in recognition of the potentially untoward effects. My job included an important nursing care intervention – to provide a therapeutic environment for healing. For instance, our cardiac care unit was a quieter environment than the surgical intensive care unit. This was intentionally done to reduce unnecessary stimulation or stress, and to facilitate the rest and healing of the heart muscle. We also gave back rubs to promote relaxation for the patients. This parasympathetic enhancing philosophy of healing seemed to disappear during the following decade as the fledgling stages of the 'move-them-in move-them-out' era began with mandated shorter 'length of stay' in hospitals.

Medical advances and changes were happening quickly. We were being taught on-the-job by doctors about new procedures, technology, medications, side effects, rationales, interventions and precautions. It was an exciting time for learning and growing professionally. However, by the late eighties, something happened to our job and nursing care. Our verbal end of shift report changed drastically. It became less about the patient still in need of their evening back rub and their toleration of the life-impact of their MI (myocardial infarction). Rather, it was more of an alphabet soup kind of lingo. This is how it went:

> "Mr. Jones, 55 y/o male, is 2 days s/p MI and CABG x2 post failed PTCA, for a 90% LAD, incisions clear, weaned off peep and extubated today, I/S is 1000, A-line wave is dampened, CO, MAP SVR all WNL."

The report contained necessary technical and physical assessment information, but the essence of it was different. I noticed the more medically advanced the patient's situation and treatment became, the less our nursing report was about the person-hood of the patient and actual nursing interventions. In the years since, the progressive introduction of more technology brought with it alarms and idiosyncrasies that continue to compete with patients for a nurse's attention.

Alarming for Nurses

Your inner call light got your attention, whatever the reason. You are experiencing job stress, frustration and even a sense of powerlessness. With reflection, you may find there were contributing events throughout your nursing career that may be key to understanding the groundswell that is continuing to build. Nurses are generally more interested in the patient, nursing care and the safe, efficient delivery of medical treatments than the business and politics of healthcare. I make no claim of expertise in either of the latter, but I feel it may be worth nurses raising their awareness of these arenas. The rationale for this relates to the terrain (environment) of the healthcare which is affecting your job, experience of work and potentially undermining your well-being.

There is a palpable discordance for today's nurses within their jobs. Nurses take on hard work and emotional challenges like people breathe air. The genuine points of incongruence, disagreement, contention and pain often seem glossed over or ignored. These tensions and strains need relief because, if sustained, they will worsen – debilitating relationships and health. Addressing them in the heart activities will reveal cues for understanding, which can create a sensed reduction in the grip of an issue or situation. In this way it becomes easier to deal with and allows for healing to occur.

(♥) Reflect and record in your journal any memories of potentially significant events and stressors for you that may
have contributed to the wear and tear on your well-being.
Include attitudes, relationships, physical symptoms and
feelings related to compassion, fatigue and burn-out. This
may shed light on the environment of your job and any
call for attention or positive action.

If terrain is a most important, determining aspect of health, you cannot affect desired change without related personal awareness and knowledge. This is what you will do in the chapters and activities gathering information from your experience and environment, both internal and external, to increase your awareness.

Financial Environment: Cost vs. Value

"Nurses are the biggest expense in healthcare." Those dissonant words echoed through me as I tried to understand if the instructor was pro nurses or against. It was 1983, when I endured the required *U.S. Healthcare Systems* class as part of my junior year nursing program curriculum. She had just highlighted a demerit that nurses unknowingly bear to this day and may still sense when they feel unappreciated. I remember asking one of my first employers, "Why don't you charge for the care that nurses provide?" They answered, "We do. We bundle it into the room charge." When nurses do not feel valued in their jobs it could be, in part, they sense their appointed place amidst the rank of rising healthcare costs, right along with necessities like pillows, blankets and air conditioning.

During the first two decades of the twenty-first century, healthcare costs became intensively scrutinized for containment, while reimbursements were tied to quality of outcomes and customer (patient) satisfaction. These customer service and outcome-related issues have commanded the attention of healthcare providers because they involve their financial bottom line. It was during this time that the job descriptions for nurses morphed again, with nurses additionally acting as technology and data entry specialists, and agents of hospitality and customer service. HCAHPS (Hospital Consumer Assessment of Healthcare Providers and Systems) and patient satisfaction survey results prove that nurses are key to patient satisfaction. Customer service in healthcare presents an almost paradoxical situation for nurses because hospitals are not hotels. According to Alexandra Robbins, journalist and author of *The Nurses: A Year of Secrets, Drama, and Miracles With the Heroes of the Hospital*, " a misguided attempt to improve healthcare has led some hospitals to focus on making people happy, rather than making them well."[3]

The value of nurses and their care is becoming more clear as it is becoming an endangered resource. Nursing care and quality have a direct effect on patient outcomes. For instance, research shows that "quality nursing care leads to improved patient outcomes."[4] Further fragmentation of the time and attention of a nurse at the bedside risks reducing outcomes. A nurse's education level has been identified as another key factor. Researchers acknowledge and validate the value of competent and compassionate care provided by all nursing staff despite the level of education or credential. However, "a higher percentage of nurses with a baccalaureate or higher correlates with better patient outcomes in hospitals"[5] including "lower congestive heart failure mortality, decubitus ulcers, failure to rescue, and postoperative deep vein thrombosis or pulmonary embolism and shorter length of stay."[6]

With the higher level of education, nurses are "better prepared to fulfill leadership and management roles and contribute to a safer work environment. They are more satisfied with their careers, which leads to lower turnover rates. These benefits translate to savings and improved staffing coverage for healthcare facilities."[7] These findings support the recommendation of "The Future of Nursing" report for nurses to increase their education levels. [8, 9]

Unstable Environment

There are serious conditions converging to form an unstable environment which significantly impacts healthcare and nurse's work:

1. The Baby Boomer Generation
2. Chronic and Debilitating Diseases
3. Nurse Shortages
4. Nurses are Stressed and Unwell
5. Lack of Preparation

The Baby Boomer Generation

The Baby Boomer Generation comprised the largest population boom in the United States, numbering 78 million births in a bell curve from 1946 to 1964. These "Boomers" represent the largest and most economically impactful group of people in America. As they were born and grew up, Boomers defined markets and influenced social change not only because of their number but also their choices and preferences. They contribute to more than half of all consumer spending. The frontrunners of the bolus turned 65 years old in 2011 and their cohorts will continue to reach that age marker until about 2029. The medical system is feeling the leading edge of this momentous wave, which challenges them to prepare for an expected onslaught of cancer, Alzheimer's, chronic disease, age-related disability and emergencies.

Chronic and Debilitating Diseases

Chronic disease, defined by the U.S. National Center for Health Statistics as a disease lasting three months or longer,[10] and debilitating diseases are the second variable. The diseases identified above are rampant and gaining a stronghold on ranks of the Boomers by compromising people's health.[11] Sixty percent of Americans have a chronic disease and forty percent have two or more.[12] According to the Almanac of Chronic Disease, older adults are more likely to have chronic diseases, but these conditions can occur at any age. As of 2004, chronic diseases were already the leading cause of death in the United States. Caregivers, whether lay or professional, bear the weight of providing for these people – emotionally, socially, and sometimes financially. The burden is consuming of their health. It is easy to see that for both segments of the population, increased healthcare needs and spending will result. The blame for the expected continued increase in healthcare costs lies with the increasing prevalence, complicated disease trajectories, and treatment intensity. Prior to dropping out of the workforce, people working with these progressively debilitating illnesses with have more sick-time use. Even while on the job, these workers may be less productive – often called "presenteeism" – which causes increased economic burden for employers.[13]

Nurse Shortages

In that same U.S. Healthcare Systems class, they taught me several statistics that were impressive, but I had little idea of their long-term value. Shortages of nurses and schools to educate them have been a recurrent plague that rears up yet again as the third variable in today's perfect storm. The most current count at the time of my class revealed there were 1.2 million nurses in the U.S. They expected that amount to double by the year 2000, maintaining nurses as the largest group of workers in the healthcare system. In fact, when we crossed the millennium, we were just about on target reaching 2.2 million nurses in 2001.

As of 2013, the World Health Statics Report accounted 29 million nurses and midwives worldwide. Of that, there were about 3.6 million nurses in the U.S. These numbers correlates with the continued and increasing integral nature of nurses in the medical care of patients regardless how much technology is in use. In fact, there was a call for a million more nurses in the U.S. by 2020.[14] Optimistically, the job outlook for registered nurses through 2028 is expected to increase at a rate much faster than the average of 12%.[15] But Boomer nurses will be retiring. There is already a shortage of nurses, nursing instructors and space in nursing education programs for students. This compounds the challenge that lies ahead for adequate staffing of nurses. Are you part of or following the Boomer generation? What is the state of your health, lifestyle and their trajectory? Are you prepared to work faster, harder and more mechanistically as a nurse? Can you feel the increasing weight you may be expected to bear? This likely means even more work-related stress.

But there is a fourth and even more concerning issue involving you, a nurse already showing signs of stress. This, unforeseen in my class thirty-five-plus years ago, is still likely not adequately accounted for.

Nurses are Stressed and Unwell

"In every category other than smoking, the health of nurses is worse than that of the average American. According to the Bureau of Labor Statistics, registered nurses have the fourth highest rate of injuries or illness on the job of all professions – even construction workers. The often 24/7 demands faced by nurses on the job contribute to the higher likelihood of nurses being overweight, having greater stress, and getting less than the recommended amount of sleep."[16] Further, Pamela Cipriano, PhD RN MSN BSN, president of the American Nurses Association (ANA) says, "It's shocking... we're not as healthy as the average public... We have a much lower intake of fruits and vegetables and one of the most striking identifiers is stress – nurses reported having two times as much workplace stress as those in the average public."[17]

⊗ Does this surprise you? It may be difficult to admit, but please review and revise the list that you made in your journal about the symptoms and illnesses you are experiencing. Remember the stress survey of your colleagues. You are not alone. You can positively influence your stress and health. Being honest with yourself empowers you by learning from symptoms, recognizing options and improving ability to advocate for your benefit.

Lack of Preparation

You are feeling the impact from all of these events. Did you see this coming? Did anyone? In my mind I hear the manager from my college restaurant job preaching his *"5Ps: Prior Planning Prevents Poor Performance"*. I suggest nurses would have prepared had we known and had the influence.

Here are more predictions that I recall from that nursing school course – a heads up for your health, career and lifestyle choices. Should they take place, they may present as further upheaval in the system or as compensatory developments following the other critical circumstances:

- Kaiser Permanente will be the model for the future of healthcare as a Health Maintenance Organization (HMO).
- Hospitals will become smaller and hi-tech for the most acute and critical levels of intervention and care.
- There will be a network of community services with varying levels of skilled nursing care and patient acuity.
- Home health will become extensive and well developed.

Nurses cannot depend upon luck when caring for patients, they must anticipate and prepare. How is it that nurses were unaware and uniformed of these developments around the looming crisis? When preparing for impact, you must take care of yourself. Even on an airplane, you're instructed to put your own oxygen mask on first. So, sisters and brothers, even though you think you do not have the time in your schedule, you must do for yourself what you need to do to build more sustainable health, renew your energy, and regain clarity, so you can be there for others.

⊗ This is a good place to make notes in your journal about insights, reactions, thoughts, questions, comments, emotions, and any solutions that come into your mind as you realize you couldn't prepare nor were you given the outlook for today's circumstances. Then consider that on a daily basis in your job, you don't have time to put on your own oxygen mask. How committed you are to making a difference for yourself.

Business Environment

A colleague nurse, with top corporate level experience in the medical industry, explained it this way:

"Every time a company needs to trim back, it is never the sales and marketing people. It is always the clinical people. Those left end up with more work than they can handle, and they are scared to complain because they do not want to lose their job. Many nurses live paycheck to paycheck. This is a constant stream of stress and those working have no voice out of fear. This is the capitalism of healthcare. When fear takes over, the people become malleable to being treated any which way just so that paycheck keeps coming. Where this ends up is that the people working are stressed and there is a bitterness among them."

For your employer, you are a resource to use, an expense to control, and a risk to manage. As a staff nurse, you are in a defined role not designed for creativity but for productivity. Might that relate to why your requests, feedback and complaints often seem to fall on deaf ears? Perhaps that is why you feel you like you cannot effect a change to improve your working environment or why you do not feel supported with adequate staffing and can rarely take a break.

It seems commonplace though under-recognized that you have been uncomfortable on the job for a while. Your employer has leveraged your adaptability and resilience at work into productivity metrics. While your situational accomplishments become the new standard – often in the interest of maintaining the revenue stream that your strained efforts made possible – your health bears the hidden costs.

If the trajectory continues of increased patient load, rising acuities and tight budgets for hiring staff nurses, the stress will continue to mount. Nurses could, at a rapid pace, join the ranks of the ill as a customer of the environment that is being constructed.

(♡) Do you see a hospital or healthcare as a business? Are they operating sustainably regarding human resources and finances? What elements, philosophies, practices and principles that you are aware of are valid to maintain viability? Which ones are not? What differences do you see between a responsibly sustainable, profitable business and one that is profit-based? Can each be mission-driven? What is the relationship between mission and profits for *sustain-ability*? Are there different definitions of success for nurses and employers? If answers or ideas come to you, write them in your journal for future inspiration.

Patient Environment

People who enter the healthcare system to access care, appropriately called patients, enter a strange world where they must release a lot of control to others. Despite their vulnerable position and important task of regaining their own health, the system assumes they will live up to that label and *be patient*. Each person brings a unique internal environment that will interact with the environment of their role as a patient.

As it is a nightmare of every nurse to be a patient, you can empathize with the discomforts of their position. There are several books written by nurses who have been patients. The memoirs of vulnerability, feelings of being out of control, tones of caregivers' voices and feelings of isolation are painful potential reflections to relate to and become aware of. A nurse, as the patient, may anticipate the staff's jobs and feel challenged to trust the practice of others because she knows the practice from the inside. She may want to control the situation of her own care. In role-confusion, she may seem impossible to please as she feels disregarded as a member of the medical team in her passive role as the patient. Nurses as patients witness and experience many of the same vulnerabilities any patient would.

Patients notice stress in their nurse and this can weigh heavily on them. "Don't I pay enough money to be here (in the Critical Care Unit) *and* to get a new nurse every shift?" That is what a patient asked me once when I told him I would be his nurse for another eight hours. He said, "You're a good nurse, but you have already been here for eight hours. Don't you need to go home and rest?" The unit was short staffed for the next shift and overtime was a commonly used quick fix. Research shows that longer shifts lead to nurse burnout[18] and patient dissatisfaction.[19]

A patient's experience can affect his or her own stress response and healing. It can impair healing while a patient is under stress.[20,21] Patients need to be in a supportive environment to *shift* into a state of healing. Fearful thoughts cause a neurochemistry of fear. These molecules of emotion circulate and bathe every cell of the body. From here they can alter health at a cellular and even genetic level.

Nurses as Environment

Consider that as a nurse, you are an important aspect of the environment for a patient. You maintain an environment conducive to dignity, safety and healing. Nursing school taught me that therapeutic use of self,[22] therapeutic relationship[23] and active listening[24] are several of the important skills of a nurse. These are part of how you, your *being-ness*, is an environment in which a patient dwells. You have likely had many patients ask, "Will you still be my nurse?" This minor element of continuity is huge and allows them to rest, knowing that 'my nurse' will be there. You monitor and do things for them they cannot do themselves momentarily or circumstantially. When patients are overwhelmed, sedated or otherwise vulnerable, you protect them – they rest in you, in the safety net of your presence. It requires both your intention and attention to accomplish these things, and the work environment must allow and provide for you doing so.

In his book, *Nurses Know! What Happened to Health Care?*, Dr. Edward M. Pallette tells his story as a patient. He observed a very different perspective of the nurses he usually worked with as colleagues. Watching them active in the trenches, he could see they were stressed. He experienced the vulnerability of being a patient, especially with a busy nurse. He interviewed nurses to find out what they knew about the situation in healthcare in 2001. Rebecca S. Ferguson, RN. contributed, "Nursing is a field, like being a mom. You have to be self-motivated to pat yourself on the back. I'm not saying you don't get that, but you will not get a lot of money or certificate awards – not a lot of Medals of Honor. We have to take care of each other. But I see a group of new nurses coming in and sometimes I wonder if the soul of nursing is missing there."[25]

In what ways are you the keeper of a safe and healing space for your patients? How do you feel as you read your colleagues' statement above? How do you think healthcare is working? What do you think has happened to healthcare? Have you felt or wondered if there is something different in the way nurses are being trained or treated in their jobs? How do you see your job description and employer expectations?

How do you feel acknowledgement and support for the value of the nurse-patient relationship? How does nursing practice policy change take place in your organization? In what ways does your manager listen, advocate and empower you and your colleagues? How does she fail? What ideas do you have about reasons for why or why not? How do you and your colleagues support and take care of yourselves and each other? How can you improve? In what ways could these relationships offer dignity for each other?

Make notes in your journal of what you discover and want to consider more deeply. Any of these related to your stress may be useful to work with as you go through the AH SUCCESS Process in Part Two.

Hostile Work Environment

An unfortunate situation occurred in 2017 when a nurse at a Utah hospital got caught in jurisdiction confusion. She seemed centered and calm while communicating with an officer about the hospital policy for drawing blood from a patient when sedated and unable to give consent. They arrested her for protecting her patient. In the online video, she appeared exemplary in holding a safe environment for her vulnerable patient. I mention this to highlight another facet of the environment that nurses work in and the potential for escalated stress faced while doing their job the way they know is best for their patients. ABC news called her act heroic. After the officers released her, she expressed that she "felt betrayed." This expresses a deep violation of the respect, trust and safety that every nurse needs to do what she feels is necessary for the best interest of her patient.[26]

To this point, in recent years, hospitals have been training staff and nurses about workplace hostility, managing combative patients, family members and active shooters. Other common areas of workplace hostility that may be more insidious include harassment, bullying and discrimination between co-workers and by managers. These are deeply disturbing and strikingly in conflict with the concepts of teamwork and employee appreciation commonly listed in values-statements and advertising.

The occurrence of any hostility-related circumstances are unimaginable where patients should improve their health and nurses are vitally imperative to that outcome. "The key to resilience in the situation is to understand the character of what is going on," says Michael Traynor in his evidence-based book, *Critical Resilience for Nurses.*[27] He further says, "… workplace bullying is unacceptable… does not cast your character… [or] your competence into doubt… [and] you do not have to justify yourself morally." Though it is often people's first reaction to resign, Mr. Traynor says, "It is far better for self-esteem to challenge and stand up."

🐘 Consider your workplace environment and any situations where the "character of what is going on" is not clear. Note these in your journal for review and consideration. Subtle actions such as labeling a nurse as "slow" can be construed as hostile in certain circumstances, particularly if she is over the age of forty. Reflect on coworkers who have left and consider their exit in the light of a potential hostile work environment being a potential cause of their resignation. Note any insights in your journal, and your answers for the questions below.

How were you affected by their situation and departure? How was the team, unit or patients affected? How do you experience the thought it could have been a retaliatory or discriminating situation? Is there any way to have stuck together with that colleague? How does the environment and culture allow or disallow this camaraderie?

Is it hostile to not provide relief for nurses to take breaks? Is it hostile to require nurses' annual vacation requests a year in advance, but withhold approval until two weeks prior to the date?

Consider keeping a journal of situations and incidents that will help you process the issues and log the details as you embark upon self-reflection and problem-solving for your stress resolution.

Addressing hostility in the workplace is a compelling and timely subject for nurses to get involved with through education and intervention. In a 2007 article in *Journal of Advanced Nursing, Debra Jackson, et. al. confirm,* "There is a clear need for nurses to develop resilience to positively overcome the professional obstacles the health care system and workplace pose on them."[28] Interventions for a nurse to consider beyond immediate self-care and relationship-based communication may necessitate using your chain-of-command, security department, incident reports, employee assistance programs, abuse and professional organizations, unions, and legal consultants.

Stereotypes in the Work Environment

Stereotypical generalizations can become a judgmental basis for biases where societies, cultures, organizations, and people get stuck. They contribute to workplace stress for nurses through the far-reaching effects of inequality, including prejudice and discrimination.[29] According to the United Nations, Human Rights Division, "Harmful stereotypes can be both hostile/negative (e.g., women are irrational) or seemingly benign (e.g., women are nurturing)."[30] There is a dominant and recessive dynamic skewed by ego, economics or influence.

Awareness of stereotypes has increased and is of broader scope than the prominent and oversimplified polarity present when my career began. The profession and employers still required nurses to wear white dresses, but we were trying to liberate from the little white caps and the custom of giving up our chairs to doctors who were typically men. In a predominantly patriarchal business and medical environment, with a primarily female workforce, there were strong gender inequalities. However, male nurses did not have their own lockers rooms in some workplaces, so they had to yield to the predominant culture. The cliché of male vs. female perspective is not one of being 'better' than the other but rather 'different', meritable and complementary.[31] Often, harm occurs in both directions.

Despite an organic history of being healers, cultivators, and wisdom-filled, women, nurses and yin practices have long been perceived and treated as recessive in healthcare and business environments. "We're the largest workforce in healthcare, but we have the smallest voice in healthcare decision making," shared Kelley Rieger, a nurse practitioner for 20 years, referring to women in nursing, in an interview with *Fast Company*.[32] The Coalition for Better Understanding of Nurses seems to concur when it related that "nurses are ignored by the media [with] only two percent of health articles use[ing] nurses as expert sources."[33]

An individually significant and economically impactful issue can be the challenging ability for a nurse to provide for herself and her family. Career mobility and gender pay inequity persist[34] as "male RNs out-earned female RNs across settings, specialties, and positions with no narrowing of the pay gap over time."[35]

The gender stereotypes and inequities are magnified when paired with other characteristics such as race, creed and color, and things like age, weight, hair color, tattoos and use of technology. There are also nursing-specific characterizations that are insidious and dangerous such as: women's work, angel, handmaiden, naughty, sexy or mean.[36]

The gender issue is dramatic because it could be considered containing any of the other minority aspects. Yet, in stark contrast, women are not a minority in healthcare. If the inequity and stereotypes are looked at as symptoms, then what are the deeper issues and causes?

> What stereotypes or inequities have you faced as a nurse? What opportunities have you passed up to address these issues? In what ways have you quietly consented to the perpetuation of a stereotype, prejudice or inequity? How will you handle similar situations moving forward? Write about your thoughts on these important questions.

This is a sensitive matter and while it may unintentionally not be comprehensive, I have not meant to exclude or exemplify any one person or perspective. Learn with every thought and interaction to be more open-minded and -hearted because it takes a rainbow of color to make sunlight.[37] This suggests that unity and wholeness comprises all that makes us unique and that working together can shine a light on previously unforeseen solutions.

Today, there is an acknowledged need for women in business and an active call for nurses to be on boards, collaborating alongside physicians on the restructuring of healthcare.[38] This presents opportunities for upward and outward job mobility. In Chapter 3 we'll look at why it is an imperative to introduce feminine principles into these traditionally masculine roles.

Environmental Background Stressors

We have looked at a web of potential environmental contributions to stress in the milieu of your work as a nurse. However, on deeper investigation, there are causes of job stress that easily go unnoticed or are generally accepted as the norm because they are in the background.

These are examples of background stressors:

- lighting and glare
- electromagnetics
- noise
- radiation
- uncomfortable or non-ergonomic furniture and equipment
- technology
- poor ventilation

- chemical exposure
- delayed bodily elimination
- missed rest and meal breaks
- lack of hydration
- temperature regulation of the environment
- proximity of co-workers
- space that is inadequate or cluttered

These elements can contribute to fatigue, frustration, inefficiency, and strain. In a single-room outpatient infusion unit where I worked, the noise level was increasing proportionate to the increase in our patient census and acuity. We were busier, patients were sicker, and we found that the noise level was distracting and becoming a burden.

Our individual verbalized concerns, disregarded by our manager, yet validated amongst ourselves, had actual effects and something needed to be done. A cacophony of staff, visitor, and patient voices from phone and in-person conversations largely created the noise in an effort to override the many other sources. Among these were phones ringing, machines working, alarming pumps, packages being opened, papers crinkled, laundry and supply stocking, patient's personal devices and TVs. The uncarpeted floor magnified the noise, as did the distress signals inside ourselves while trying to cope.

We endured in a somewhat dis-empowered manner because our dismissed voices became more like persistent nagging complaints. Unfortunately, this can often happen when nurses try to speak up. We had much responsibility and were too busy to build a focused effort of influence that stated what we needed. Eventually, we inspired investigation. Our manager shared the findings of the 'noise level' study. While it changed nothing noticeable in our work environment, the shocking results below validated our complaints.

According to the National Institute on Deafness and Other Communication Disorders, they state the following measurements in decibels:

140 dB	Jet plane
125 dB	Threshold for pain begin
95 dB	Arc welding « **This is where our unit scored**
85 dB	Hearing damage begins with prolonged, eight-hour exposure
80 dB	Average city traffic
70 dB	Below 70 is safe for hearing
50-60 dB	A quiet office
20 dB	A whisper
10 dB	Normal breathing

It is common to adapt to background stress through desensitization. While it may be protective of your sanity to filter out excessive noise and stimuli, in your job it's dangerous to become desensitized. Alarm fatigue is a specific related phenomenon which raises a major concern. Research reveals it occurs because of sensory overload and overwhelm and it threatens your health, job and patient safety.

   List the background stress you endure in your workplace in the order that they come to you. Rate each from 1 to 5 for the level of stress it causes you using five for the most intolerable. Write the number beside each item on your list. Contemplate the impact of these on you, and any actions you may take to address them and their impact.

Burnout Environment

In April 2019, the World Health organization made "burn-out" an official medical diagnosis. Many doctors say a toxic work environment is one of the biggest contributing factors to burn-out.[39] It has its own identifying number in the *International Classification of Disease manual, Eleventh Revision (ICD-11)*[40] under "problems related to employment or unemployment". It is diagnosable only as "phenomena in the occupational context" and is "characterized by three dimensions":

1. Feelings of energy depletion or exhaustion,
2. Increased mental distance from one's job, or feelings of negativism or cynicism related to one's job; and
3. Reduced professional efficacy.

This concept is of no surprise to nurses who have talked and joked about burnout for decades.[41] Nurses want a collaborative and caring employer. They have not spoken up because of the risk of job loss or the derogatory implication of failure. With this 'it's about time' recognition of a serious problem, the term might be more accurate as 'burned-up' from a functional perspective, because it is more likely a resulting symptom of environmental issues that took their toll on the well-being of the nurse.[42]

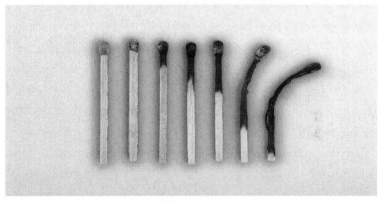

Photo licenced from AdobeStock / beeboys

It is important to distinguish between compassion fatigue and burnout. Burnout tends to be chronic and generalized, while compassion fatigue is acute and involves compassion and empathy.[43] They share similar symptoms, so medically they may be treated the same. However, because of the unique causes, the way to address restoring well-being for each should be different. In either cause, self-care and regulation are imperative. Positive action for success must include interventions that balance and correct the root causes which may include professional guidance or changing environments such as your workplace.

What is coming up for you? Refer to your lists of background stress and environmental stressors, and your list of symptoms of stress that you have written in your journal. Does changing your perspective of them to that of being symptoms of a deeper, maybe environmental issue, open the possibility of a different understanding? Where does this possibility lead you? What are your thoughts and reactions to the new "burn-out" diagnosis? You may recognize shades of grief, loss, remorse, betrayal or self-neglect. Are you ready to get in line for a leave of absence? Are you willing to *shift* this experience using self awareness?

You will learn ways to change your relationship with and experience of stress in chapters to come. Write as much as you feel moved to in your journal about these concepts. It is okay to purge your emotions, feelings and thoughts by putting them in writing in your journal.

The environment of healthcare seems to be cortisol-laden where practitioners take a lot of risks and their patients risk a lot for a chance at regaining health. There is pain, trauma, and loss. Nurses are tired, overburdened with tasks, and need a break. Nurses burn out while managers bear down on productivity. "Impact of Workplace Climate on Burnout Among Critical Care Nurses in the Veterans Health Administration," an article published in *Critical Care Nurse* magazine, presents research conclusions suggesting "in efforts to reduce burnout, emphasis should be placed on improving local workplace climate."[44]

Environmental Incongruence

If you have done shift-work (external environment), which is common for nurses, you know well that one of the common related stressors is the chaotic sleep-wake cycle (internal environment). It will not surprise you that researchers have found that "an out-of-phase circadian rhythm [internal environment] is a health hazard."[45] This is a potent environmental incongruence in healthcare that needs to be acknowledged and granted sincere, creative intervention. Any stress can cause biorhythmic disharmony which can causes sleep disruption and lead to similar conditions.

Brace yourself for the next bit of news. Dieter Kunz, director of the Sleep Research and Clinical Chronobiology Research Group at Charité–Universitätsmedizin Berlin, calls shift workers "a model for internal desynchronization."[46] This is because shift workers are known to have increased morbidity and mortality for a diseases including cardiovascular disorders and cancer. In 2007 the World Health Organization decreed that shift work is a risk factor for breast cancer, which led to the compensation of some female shift workers with breast cancer. Denmark started the compensation of female shift workers with breast cancer after the 2007 World Health Organization decree.

Do you see business as competitive? How so or not? What about healthcare? List your examples. What competition is there in your job as a nurse? Do men and women differ in their competitiveness? What qualities do each display that are competitive? Are spite, jealousy, gossip, and not speaking up competitive? How do these qualities mix with the competitive elements of business? How do you respond to an environment that creates competition between nurses? Describe the environment that it creates.

Does the business side of healthcare – to be faster, do more with fewer resources and win performance merit – affect your caring for patients? If so, how? By what means can you be honest with yourself and colleagues about the qualities of personality and elements of your job you thought of or wrote, but are not proud of? Can nurses better manage stress and encourage growth in each other as individuals and leaders, perhaps even influence policy and system change? If you have impulses, ideas, questions, and action-items come up for you, write them in your journal for consideration.

If it is common employer-practice to overlook rest breaks and deny time off, how does a nurse get replenished? In the early years of my career, nurses could use sick leave for a "personal day" at some hospitals. Today some employers scrutinize use of sick days and issue demerits in annual evaluations.

You and your colleagues know firsthand the effects of adrenaline and cortisol. These are the main hormones your body makes for your survival of nearly every workday. Excluding the urgencies and emergencies, it will take self-aware and health-aware nurses innovating together, to be an influence toward a thriving work environment. Our innovative discussion about the importance of environment in your well-being finds support in the conclusions of a 2009 *Health Affairs* study: "Improving nurses' work environments, including nurse staffing, may improve the patient experience and quality of care."[47] That is the success that you are looking for – to thrive with health in all areas of your life – including your career. There is a dynamic relationship between internal and external environments to explore which will facilitate your achievement.

CHAPTER 3

INTERNAL AND EXTERNAL ENVIRONMENT

Some perceptions of stress are general, but most are circumstantial. What is stressful for one may present a welcomed challenge for another. Yogi and Indian monk, Paramahansa Yogananda teaches the circumstances of one's environment are made up of an outer and inner world. The first engaging in action and interaction, the second determines your happiness or unhappiness.[1] Therefore, it is imperative to give attention to learning about yourself, your internal environment, and relationship with what appears to be external.

As a new grad nurse, cardiology fascinated me and I diligently learned the medical-side of nursing for cardiac patients. Working with cardiac patients motivated me to learn how I could maintain my health and avoid getting heart disease. I was inspired to change my diet, meditate and continue the dedicated exercise routine I started in college. I also taught my patients about self-care and lifestyle choices because I learned that taking care of health *proactively* is the best way to maintain it and facilitate restoring it.

One patient I remember well is John, a sixty-two year-old businessman-turned-cardiac-patient. He liked to tease about the inscription – Young, RN – on my hanging nurse's watch pinned to my scrub top. "Just how young are you?" he'd joke. I was 20, which was young for having completed 4 years of nursing school.

He had several realizations after learning and doing relaxation breathing and visualization. Immediately, he put aside his inner-skeptic when he found that he enjoyed doing them. He was surprised that he could observe his own breathing, something he never previously noticed. His big realization was that he often gulped for air or held his breath while engaged in business-related activities. He figured out, breathing that way was a habit because of stress, so he did not realize he was having significant shortness of breath leading up to his heart attack. He was amazed he missed the clues. He said breathing deeply provided a refreshing break because it also quieted his usual mental noise and strife.

To calm his internal milieu, he described the visualization that worked for him vividly: *I'm wearing my lucky green-plaid golf shorts and white polo. My buddies and I got the first tee time of the day — he course is ours to conquer. I feel limber, relaxed, and fill my lungs with cool morning air. A smooth wind up and swoosh, a perfect swing on exhale, crack and I ride the ball (my favorite moment) as it sails toward the green for my hole-in-one.*

His heart rate would noticeably decrease on the cardiac monitor while he did this.

Collectively, my cardiac patients revealed similar truths about their lives, jobs, perceptions, and experiences. They told me they felt like something was chasing them in life. They needed to be successful and to get ahead. There was a race they were engaged in and they were uncertain why, but they felt an urgency and pressure to take part with intensity. Their external environment with the demands of their jobs dominated over their personal lives. They had less time, patience and attention for their home-life, family, hobbies, themselves or to spend in nature. I taught them, as I did John, to use body awareness to monitor how they were doing amidst the stressful external environment and to use relaxation breathing to ease the tension they experienced inside their mind and body.

How do you relate to the feelings the experiences of these people? What associations or similarities do you notice between how you feel on the inside and how your day seems to go? How are you affected by your surroundings and the conditions in your workplace environment? What are common environmental stressors for you, including while at work? When was the last time you spent an hour or more in nature? How do you experience being in nature? How is that experience different for you from being inside a building? Allow yourself to explore freely your perceptions, experience and effects within your life.

Record any motivations for improvement or change. Commit to spending ten minutes each workday in nature – easy enough to do if you take your break. Notice any differences after doing this the first time. What effects do you experience in your internal milieu after a week of doing this? After a month?

Sometimes I removed my footwear as I left work and walked barefoot in the grass patches on the way to my car. I found this to be amazing for my tired feet, body and mind. From behind one day I heard, "That looks like it feels good." The man in scrubs took his shoes off and, as the grass cooled his feet, he let out a major sigh and said, "I needed this." We could not contain our hearty bubbles of laughter as we mused at the simplicity and effectiveness of being barefoot in the grass to neutralize the effects of our stressful workday.

Going barefoot and being in nature are basic needs and natural instincts for me. However, while writing the second edition of this book I read of a recently discovered medical breakthroughs related to "Earthing". An article in the Journal of Environmental and Public Health states, "…emerging scientific research has revealed a surprisingly positive and overlooked environmental factor on health: direct physical contact with the…surface of the Earth…[and that] modern lifestyle separates humans from such contact."[2] Does this surprise you? Do this for yourself soon and often. Try walking barefoot or lying on the ground to connect with the Earth. The effect is like that of a potent antioxidant. "Reconnection with the Earth's electrons has been found to promote intriguing physiological changes and subjective reports of well-being… including better sleep and reduced pain."[3]

Society vs. Nature

In an open-air class held at the yoga pavilion above the turquoise waters of the Caribbean Sea, one could not avoid feeling wonderful or at least in wonder. The economist John Perkins spoke to the attendees of the holistic educational retreat held by The Omega Institute on the island where I lived. Stephan Rechtschaffen, MD, the institute's cofounder, had given me the privilege of working with him as the local public relations person and faculty massage therapist. The prominent faculty member, Mr. Perkins, was also an author, environmentalist and founder of the non-profit organizations *Dream Change* and *The Pachamama Alliance*. He had done many years of volunteer and independent work in the Amazon with the Shuar Indian peoples of the area. He shared how he previously arranged for the chiefs of the Shuar to meet the chiefs in America. As they landed in Washington, DC, one chief asked, "What's wrong with the women in your society?" For them, it was clear from the air, and confirmed upon landing, that they had arrived at a place that was suffering a severe imbalance between society and nature, between the forces of masculine and feminine. Keep in mind, this is from the perspective of male individuals from a *wilder-world* seeing the *civilized* West for the first time – Shamanism not chauvinism. In contrast to their home, the Shuar chiefs saw a place, from their perspective, that suppressed nature. The unhealthy feminine expression was obvious because of the man-made structures and grid of roadways that dominated the landscape with relatively few trees or green areas remaining. For the Shuar, this served as validation for why their rainforest home was suffering destruction and ruin as Western culture encroached.

Perkins referred to a characteristic of the indigenous Shuar culture in the jungle of the Amazon – both men and women have an important presence. They practice a balance of the masculine and feminine principles inherent within their culture and society. The relationship they cultivated was one where either would temper or enhance the other rather than a dominance of one over the other. For instance, men are the hunters, but they hunt by the guidance of the women. The women observe the sun, moon, seasons, and they cultivate the garden. The women advise the men when there is plenty to eat and no longer a need for hunting. Likewise, they advise the hunters to hasten their efforts when an early or extended winter is imminent.

Are you surprised to read the Shuar's perspective of the society and culture of the West? Make notes as you answer the following questions. What is your first impression when you look at the photo of New York City and Central Park below? What similarities and contrasts do you observe? At this distance, can you tune in to the life and vitality of the city and the park and how do they compare? What qualities of stillness do you glean from the perspective of each photo? Does one feel more natural? What movement, sounds, temperature or quality of air do you sense in the city compared to the park? Does one area in the photo look more stressful or calming compared to the other?

Imagine yourself in each location and sense your experience within your body-tension, excitement, heart rate, breathing pattern, solitude. How important do you see nature to your well-being and in what ways? Do you see an imbalance of the masculine and feminine in the environment where you live? What resemblance do you see to the Shuar's perceptions? Do you see any need or purpose for the advice of the Shuar related to balancing the masculine and feminine aspects of our culture? How do you otherwise relate to the Shuar's perspective? In your journal, explore your perspective of progress and a man-made environment, including how it relates to your health and relationship with the natural world.

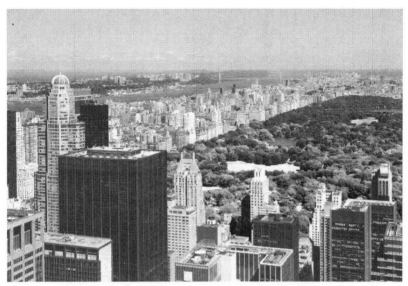

New York City, Manhattan Skyline and Central Park
Photo licensed from Adobe Stock / Andy

Perkins wrote many books on the principles for health, healing, and sustainability, inspired by the teachings of the Shuar people. The message from the Shuar to America – change the dream. "It is your people who are destroying these forests," they said. "Your oil, mining and lumber companies. Behind all that is your dream of bigger cities, higher buildings, and more cars. Go back to your people and help them change their dream."[4]

The dream comes from within. It represents our internal environment, but profoundly influences and affects the external environment, the community, culture, and nature. Through the organization that he started in 1987, DreamChange.org, Perkins has been delivering this message and facilitating healthy change in people and communities for their health and the health of the environment and nature.

Describe your "dream" in your journal. Be deeply honest with yourself about it. This is the dream you hold as an outlook of the world that reflects your values into all that you do. After writing about it, consider what elements facilitate healthy, sustainable living and which are counter to it – driving waste, consumption, pollution, nutrient-poor eating and even your stress. How accurately does your life and world reflect your dream? Does it match the attitude you portray daily? The AH-SUCCESS Process can be applied to address the disparities.

Mind Environment

The Shuar chiefs were imparting wisdom when they said, "Change the dream." A healthy, natural external environment is imperative to our health and likewise its depletion will contribute to our ails and ills. The mindset in the West appeared to them to be about growth through man-made productivity. The successful pursuit of this *picture* resulted in what the Shuar saw – the imbalance with nature and an unsustainable relationship with dwindling natural resources, including our health. Do you see how inner and outer environments show effects resulting from each other.

How is it tolerable for life-forms to become endangered, even extinct, while our toxic waste and convenient, disposable items will never fully disappear? Did you realize at the end of 2018, life expectancy in the U.S. measurably declined? Key contributors are suicide and overdose.[5] What is the *picture* (dream) we collectively hold in our minds and hearts as a society, and how does it contribute to the above-described condition? It may be more difficult to pick these out if you are accustomed to minimal diversity. Exposure to economic, cultural, geographic or theological variations, whether through a friendship, travel or study, make it easier to reflect and contemplate such things.

Which of these might be external examples of the predominant-expressed cultural internal environment: Progress, Convenience, Growth, Winning? If you are uncertain, spend fifteen minutes in a city, a city park, and an untouched nature-area outside of town. Observe each and be aware of your experience of each. Reflect comparatively and make notes. What does the condition of nature in each of these environments suggest about the condition of our collective inner worlds of mind and health? Which also shows up in the healthcare environment that may contribute to your stress, and in what ways? What shows up within yourself as expressions of masculine and feminine? What would it be like if the masculine and feminine that exists within and without all made peace with each other? List in your journal your responses to these questions.

Regarding your work environment, what *picture* (dream) is the standard for your place of employment? One of productivity, sterility, efficiency, relaxation, comfort, vitality? How does it support your health and well-being? Even deeper, what is the picture you hold for the health of your patients? Be specific, even by diagnosis, as it may differ for myocardial infarction, diabetes or cancer. What is the picture you hold for your own health?

Answer these questions in your journal. It is important to take time to discover that *picture*, if it is not clear to you because of the inherent power of influence it holds as what the Shuar call your "dream". How does your *picture* create or limit health? Once you have learned the AH SUCCESS Process, you may come back to this list for prompts.

An amazing concept revealed in the book and in the movie, *The Secret,* is that your thoughts [internal environment] create your reality [external environment].[6] Science has further come to understand that the experiences of life are a projection of the inner *picture*, the condition or circumstances in your mind and heart. It appears *out there,* but you are seeing reflected to you what is within you. For instance, if you carry unresolved anger, it will incline you to feel threatened by and see anger in certain situations. So you may unnecessarily verbally lunge at a colleague who asks for your help because you unknowingly take it as a competitive challenge. In reverse, you may notice drivers seem aggressive around you on the road or people are short with you when you ask them a simple question. "The world sometimes shows you what you are and often shows you what you judge."[7] Will you soften any protective or defensive mindset and let that possibility sink in? This also means you can influence the interactions by changing your *dream* (picture), thoughts, emotions, and actions. Your reality will have resulting change because what you see in your mind and feel in your heart, you create.

To some this may not sound like hard science, but it is science. It is *meta,* however, meaning beyond or above; in this case, beyond the physical or material. As suggested by Paul Levy, author and founder of the *Awakening in the Dream* community in Portland, Oregon, "Meta-physical considerations are unavoidable if we are truly interested in comprehensive knowledge of the whole and not merely in practical, material concerns."[8] New scientific discoveries not yet woven into our mainstream systems and paradigms are turning things upside down and inside out, including in modern medicine. This is likely related to what you sense when you feel something is just not right or wonder if there must be something more.

Placebo Environment

A placebo effect is the change associated with a placebo – something inert and incapable of producing the effect. Historically it means 'to please' and is used in research and medicine as a neutral comparison or to placate when there is nothing else to offer. Placebo effect has been attributed to perception of the one who receives it. A placebo environment can be an internal or external environment that enhances ones' perception, usually positively else it would be called nocebo. Characteristics of the environment have been proven to influence the effects. The color and number of pills, the words, demeanor and clothing of the practitioner, route of administration and even the setting, such as whether given in a hospital or clinic, can influence the receivers' perception and effects they experience.

Harnessing the power of your thoughts and *pictures* in your mind, and internal environment is a foundational step in healing and creating well-being within yourself (empowerment) and for those in your care (influence). This is because you cannot think your way logically into healing. Though healing may seem illogical, it involves internal intelligence. One of the most impactful pieces of evidence from medical science to support the power of a person's *picture* or dream with its associated feelings, referred to as a belief, is the proven validity of the placebo effect.[9] This is how the wisdom of the internal environment of your mind can influence what materializes in your body and the external environment, such as when people told they will never walk again, walk. Athletes have greater achievements through visualization, affirmation, belief, and owning the power to create their reality, which is closely related to the power of placebo.

As a young athlete, Joe Dispenza, DC, applied his knowledge, philosophy and faith to create healing in his body of the six broken vertebrae he sustained from a car vs. bike accident during the cycling portion of a triathlon. He declined a medically recommended high-risk surgery. He committed himself to studying the process and applying the principles, and created healing in his body. He recounts, "At nine and a half weeks after the accident, I got up and walked back into my life – without having any body cast or any surgeries."[10] Today he is a thought leader, neuroscientist, and author on healing and the power of thought, including the book *You Are the Placebo*.

I remember Richard and Carol, two patients in a cancer therapy drug trial together. They quickly bonded because they were experiencing the same diagnosis. During the trial, they scheduled their treatments together and kept up with each other's appointments and results. If one was late or absent, the other would experience a deep sense of loss and concern for their absent comrade. They were in it together, for each other, and both did well through the treatment.

Upon the completion of the trial, they had a huge decision to make. It was also a very personal one. They shared their concerns about learning what medication they received because they were both doing so well without knowing. What if one had gotten the placebo? What would that mean to their outcome? They had become close friends, involved in each other's life. What if one died? Curiosity got the best of them and they found out together.

I witnessed the shattering of their *picture*. Carol had received the drug and Richard had received the placebo. Both of them were in shock. Their imagination became filled with fear and what-ifs. Carol felt guilty. Richard felt deceived. He had a few more minor challenges during the study, but overall had done extremely well. The trajectory of his health went sharply downhill in disappointment.

Carol visited the infusion center periodically to see "my nurses." It was like coming home for her because we had shared her journey and her loss. We gave encouragement, but she felt alone. She stopped coming to visit. There was no way to know how she fared. Survivor's guilt is real. The placebo effect is real. Emotions, and especially broken hearts, affect health.

In what ways do you see the powerful effects of companionship, thoughts, attitudes, feelings, emotions and beliefs for Carol and Richard? Have you witnessed the placebo effect in a patient? Review the disparity in the scenario between their presentation and your thoughts and feelings, confusion or judgements. Were you able to accept their reality even though you could not validate it conventionally? Situations that involve pain and pain control are common scenarios involving nurses and patients which tread among the difficulties of validating perceptions and results.

Explore the placebo effect further in your journal, including perhaps an experience of your own power of belief and instances of the placebo effect. This may be difficult to recall or admit because it seems to resemble the conventional dismissive diagnostic comment, "It's all in your head." Being honest with yourself will acknowledge the power of your beliefs.

Lissa Rankin, MD, says, "...the scientific community, medical establishment has been proving for over fifty years that the mind can heal the body...we call it the placebo effect and we've been trying to outsmart it for decades. ...trying to bring in new treatments [and] new surgeries into the medical establishment..."[11] If you want to ally with the power of the placebo, you must be willing to work with your mind, thoughts and perceptions, and accept that power can be used to self propel and to self sabotage. A nocebo effect may be in play with clichés such as, "You're your own worst enemy" and "You just need to get out of your own way." Herein lies potential empowerment for dealing with your stress and related symptoms.

There is an edge of this placebo thing that is uncomfortable. It can easily be challenged as a cultural myth that you can or must *fight* illness or stress with positive thinking. The experience of this *new-age guilt* results from the perception that one has *failed* if they get stressed, ill or do not become well again. Conventional science has yet to calculate how much self responsibility we have. It is new and perhaps disturbing to consider the potential sphere of influence positive thinking could exhibit when our norm, as the Shuar suggest, is to think that we take part in a disconnected culture. Within the same concept though, it is likely in your favor to be open to the possibility that you take part in creating your experiences, subtly and profoundly, long before you (or science) can detect it visibly, physically or tangibly. Skills helpful with intentional positive thinking, awareness, openness, forgiveness, and trust relate to *response-ability*, and are part of the AH SUCCESS Process. Your awareness of the placebo effect is an initial step toward intentionally working with this force.

Imagine a small community hospital where staff and patients are familiar and on a first name basis. The decor is colorful, the overall atmosphere is personal, comforting and homelike. Notice how this description makes you feel. Compare that with the environment of a larger institution with more standardized decor, more anonymity, and a technological or corporate approach. Imagine being there and notice how this makes you feel. Make notes about any differences between the two environments especially related to the morale of nurses, camaraderie between units, patient satisfaction, and the experience of stress, emotions and symptoms for each. What environmental placebos or nocebos do you perceive in these scenarios? Make notes about any realizations you have, particularly if they relate to your stress and job.

Nurses who have worked in a community hospital that was purchased by a larger healthcare organization can easily recount the changes that occurred in the work environment, relationships, experience of work, and the patient's experience of care. This occurrence can bring on stress, anxiety, *shifts* in morale and more.[12] A large more sophisticated hospital can bring new technology and wider treatment options and can serve more people. It begs an answer to the riddle… which is better? There are gains and losses with each. It is about perspective. Some of your answers may have to do with people being the blood and backbone of care. Mechanizing or managing nursing into an assembly-line type of practice counters the fact that nurses are the conduit of care. While a nurse's health and well-being are within her power and self *response-ability*, the organization must also value and promote both. A nurse is a vital placebo suggestion of well-being and safety to a vulnerable patient,

Interactive Environments

Are you seeing the interweave of environments? How can they not influence one another? Do you see that your inner environment is fundamental to how you react to, interact with, or influence the external environments? The job of your mind is to make associations. This means it is important to examine and find space between your tightly held assumptions, associations, rationales, and reasonings which can close off your mind to opportunities. From where you are now, get to know your self and your mind by looking within and getting beyond any limiting beliefs you can identify. This will 'un-cloud' your perception so you can know yourself better by seeing more clearly what is true within yourself versus the fearful and un-serving ideas about yourself. Meditation can assist you with knowing yourself in this way and discerning what is true for you and what is an external influence. In this book you will experience several mediations and will find more information about meditation under resources at the end of the book.

How did we develop such culturally limited and self-defeating thinking when there is innate intelligence in our bodies always creating health? When humans culturally became distant from nature, they became cut off from a vast source of information. We are not born with instructions to operate our body or a manual for how to navigate life. Because of the extent to which emotions continue to be down-played, it further significantly reduces our self-knowledge. So each individual must ask and seek to know. There are teachings from ancient cultures that offer guidance. There are also modern scientific discoveries that provide confirmation and new knowledge. Collectively they provide a more wholistic understanding.

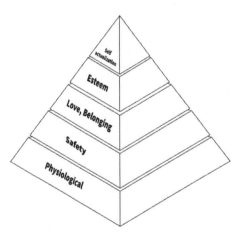

Maslow's pyramid showing hierarchy of needs.
Image licensed from Adobe Stock / EvgeniyBobrov

Do you recall Maslow's hierarchy of needs? It depicts human needs in a pyramid, with physiological needs at the broad-based foundational bottom where we all start our climb through life. Maslow's hierarchy suggests that as we attain the externally focused accomplishments, we will eventually arrive at self-actualization at the relatively distant and tiny top of the pyramid. "Self-actualization, according to Maslow, represents growth of an individual toward fulfillment of the highest needs – those for meaning in life, in particular."[13]

From this, perspective, personal and worldly growth is linear and sequential. Our internal environment then, culturally evolves under the heavy influence of staying in line, following in order, seeking external reward and accomplishment – before knowing our intrinsic value. Unfortunately, this perspective of competing for basic needs and approval, feeds insecurity and perceived inequity because it undermines belonging and self-worth. This is a place where we humans get stuck, with many potential points for disappointment, judgement, societal labelling. How many people do you know who have eaten, clothed and shopped their way to happiness and self-actualization? Do you sense an 'upside down-ness' that makes it culturally more acceptable to compete and be in the struggle to have our physical needs met than to share and flourish together in the life-enhancing abundance and actualization?

> In your journal draw a basic snowman before reading
> further. What did you draw? Do you feel as if you did what
> I asked? Did you do it right? Three circles on top of each
> other, smallest on the top and largest on the bottom? Did
> you add charcoal eyes and carrot nose too? Finish your
> snowman however you wish before reading further.
>
> How creative did you get, once you had permission? Did
> you draw a cowboy hat and chaps or a pirate hat an eye
> patch? I gave you permission to finish it as you wish. It can
> be difficult to color outside of the lines, so to speak, when
> you were taught to follow, please others, and get it right. If
> you want to draw another snow-person go ahead, unleash
> your creativity – how about one with a hula skirt? Write
> what you learned about your inhibitions, creativity, rules,
> permissions, courage and other ways.

Many great minds and successful people have shared their secrets for internal environment success through "fulfillment of the highest needs – those for meaning in life" which defy the ordered principles of the pyramid. Dale Carnegie, Napoleon Hill, Viktor Frankl, Epictetus and Einstein are a few.[14] Their teachings and writings similarly mention self-awareness, self knowledge, and self-worth. These are necessary prior to accessing innate gifts of meaning, inner vision, and wisdom. It is by harnessing the power of your thoughts, attitudes and beliefs, and through visualization that manifestation and higher-level needs are realized.

Knowing self-value leads to the certainty that "a candle loses nothing by lighting another candle" while everyone gets warm and shares in the brighter light.[15] *Living* these inner truths *is* their *actualization* through your actions. Can you see how inner value influences external environment in a culture, workplace or society? This supportive way seems to ease the scarcity and competition dilemmas of the pyramid of needs. With this as a new cultural norm from birth – to create and ensure belonging and high esteem – it promotes cooperative relationship and balances safety needs while tending to physiological necessities.

Self-actualization involves heart-based living. This is the true nature of the health and success that you desire, for harmonious interaction between your internal and external environments. You have surely seen someone looking radiant and harmonious – they exude health. What is it that turns that on? I am suggesting to you that it is heart, and the joy and love within it.

In his book, *The Hidden Messages in Water*, Dr. Masaru Emoto, showed that the structure of water changed according to the quality of human thought he exposed it to. The crystal patterns seen in frozen water after exposed to loving thoughts and words were intricately beautiful, while exposure to negativity produced asymmetrical, fractured and clouded patterns.[16] The implications of these results for human health are stunning since water comprises much of the body. Emotions are primitive and vibrational, entraining every cell to fear or love disease or ease. This directly influences the health in our internal environment, which influence the external environment. That inner call light getting your attention now is a message from deep within your cells, heart and soul.

(♡) How is your internal environment – your deep heart – doing? What descriptive qualities or characteristics does your deep heart possess or wish to express – fatigue, pain, loss, disappointment, courage, sorrow or gratitude? These indicate healing interventions are needed. In Western medicine these fall under the psychological specialties but maybe it is becoming clearer how these cannot be solely addressed with yang treatments like medications.

Consider what you were taught in relation to the principles of survival, your needs, priorities and self expression while growing up, going to school and working in your job. Were you encouraged to get the 'right' answer or were you given opportunities to create a solution to a problem or explain your point of view? Was your benchmark to be better than the other person or be the best expression of yourself? How do you experience or feel the difference in these paired concepts?

How would life be different if you had been taught to see every challenge as a chance to become a better expression of yourself and your talents? How would life be different if you were taught you are invaluable by virtue of your birth, and your purpose is to express your value in the world? Also, that within a peculiarity that blocks and challenges, lies the alchemy of your success.[17]

How well is our current cultural dream working with consideration of these concepts? What would you like to see change? What can you do within yourself and your life to make that change? Address your pondering in your journal.

Balancing Environments

What does balance mean to you? Is it equality, symmetry or complementary? The message from the Shuar sheds light on the need to re-balance the masculine and feminine in America, as evidenced by the external environment they observed. They suggest doing so by changing our individual and collective dream, which involves the environment of our mind and heart, our relationships and our values. What they interpreted was a yang expression that dominates the culture, society and healthcare.

Hopefully, the perspective forming as you read is nothing like a 'men vs. women' paradigm. Ideally, it would be characteristic of the Chinese philosophy of Yin-Yang, associated with masculine and feminine energies, their interdependent relationship, balance, and the expression of each and together as a whole.[18]

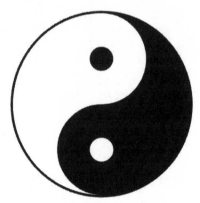

Yin-Yang. Image in public domain / Gregory Maxwell

The Yin-Yang symbol looks like two equal but opposing figures of black and white. However, Yin-Yang is not defined by gender or color. The dominant shapes are in symbiotic complement with one another. This relationship cultivates and gives rise from one to the other while the fullness of its own expression emerges and recedes in dynamic balance. Each has characteristics of the other within its expression, depicted by the dot which is the 'seed' within of the other. It is this dynamic interaction that maintains the whole – the harmony of the universe and all that is within it. This movement is life; imbalance and stagnation do not sustain health or life. It further provides for sustainability by the way they give rise to each other as they interrelate. This is a strategic aspect of this philosophy that if embraced, can bring harmony to the West, with its strain, depletion and excess. What would a balanced community of healthy people in a healthy environment look like?

Everything has a tendency toward Yin or Yang. Yet everything – nutrition, movement, solitude, work, use of resources, production of goods, giving, rest – expresses in shades of Yin and Yang. The measure of expression is by relationship. Yin is about organics, tending, preparation and cultivation. Yang is about the yield, the fruit and harvest. The businesses providing healthcare need to be fruitful (yang) to continue to provide service. However, your experience of stress proves that 'the fruit' cannot come at the health-expense of its cultivators – nurses and others – which is an unbalanced, unsustainable model of relationships.

In the first decade of this century, there was already a predicted imbalance between the looming deficit of nurses and healthcare workers with an progressively aging and ailing population. What counterbalancing measures were taken to offset or prepare? As it happened, those who are working cannot spend enough of their life force energy to make the ill patients well enough, nor the bottom line be positive enough. Improved outcomes must come from a more balanced and sustainable effort and source. Scurrying around to treat symptoms without seeking the answers to big questions, 'Why?' and 'How?' will probably only lead to more frenzy and illness. Is there a way to prevent or at least minimize the increasing prevalence and predicted extreme trajectory for illness?[19]

Write in your journal about what is coming up for you as you consider these perspectives. Do you experience a sense of ease or stress with the way of Yin-Yang? And with the Western way? Describe how the balance created and maintained with Yin-Yang compares or contrasts for you with the linear and dualistic way of opposites and competition which dominate Western culture? What correlations do you find between balance and imbalance and health and illness in your life, job, stress? Indicate which are internal and external environments. Propose how to balance them for positive outcomes.

As nursing and medicine work together in the healthcare, are they complementary or is one accessory? Now consider the relationship of medicine and nursing where nursing is yin to medicine (yang) in the Western medical model.[20,21] There is a seed of each in the other. Both care, both think, but they differ, yet complement in their way. As a nurse, your care, compassion and empathy (yin) is coupled with knowledge, discernment and leadership (yang). Can you see how nurses (yin) can gain expression from within our present day environment of the healthcare system (yang)? For instance, your strength (yang) comes from your compassion (yin). Compassion is necessary to balance the often challenging medical environment and treatments.

On a small island where I worked, there was no hospital. We provided supportive health care (yin) and emergency intervention and stabilization (yang). The nurses were independent, running the facility 24 hours per day and calling the doctors if needed. The nurses spoke up (yang) and had the doctors stand with them to stop the rental of mopeds and motor cycles because of the increase in accidents and injuries to visitors. In contrast, another more metropolitan (yang) island where I worked, solely provided mopeds and motor cycles for visitors to rent. Surgeons in the hospital worked around the clock pinning hips, grafting skin and treating head injuries (yang). Think about the balance within these two environments, services available and safety tolerance. Notice the yin and yang in dynamic interaction.

If Yin is about organics, tending, preparation and cultivation, then Yang is about the yield, the fruit and harvest. The businesses (yang) providing healthcare need to be fruitful (yang) to continue to provide service (yang). However, your stress proves that 'the fruit'(yang) cannot come at the health-expense of its cultivators (yang) – nurses and other employees – which is not a sustainable model. Can you see how this example exhibits an imbalance of yang? In the first decade of this century, there was already a predicted and looming deficit of nurses and healthcare workers, concurrent with a progressively aging and ailing population. Those who are working cannot spend enough of their life force energy to make the ill patients well enough, nor the bottom line be positive enough. Improved outcomes must come from a more balanced and sustainable effort and source.

Scurrying around to treat symptoms without seeking the answers to big questions, 'Why?' and 'How?' will probably only lead to more frenzy and illness.

Regarding Yin-Yang, how do you understand health and healthcare? What changes or balancing improvements would you like to see? How can the healthcare environment become more health promoting and life enhancing for patients, nurses and staff? What does promoting health mean to you? What does promoting health mean to you? If many chronic diseases are linked to environmental influences, lifestyle and the standard American diet (often called SAD), what effect on health would you expect from a healthy environment, lifestyle, and diet? What is a healthy environment, lifestyle and diet? With whom does the power to change lifestyle, food choices, and environmental toxin exposure lie? What ways could nurses lead this change? What balancing impact could such changes have on the outlook of current healthcare predicaments? What about your health? What does balance look like for you? Answer these important questions in your journal.

Environment of Health

In contrast to a conventional yang model of medicine focused on specialized symptom-based care, a nursing model with a theoretical basis in holism, healing and a more organic means of cultivating health, is more yin. Nurses have much to contribute in creating a culture of health within the healthcare system but also in people, lifestyles, and communities outside the system.

Bringing your energetic and healthy self to do meaningful work means you will do healthier work. How could business outcomes be different if employers listened to and provided a healthy work environment for nurses? What if that work environment included integrated rest and nutrition breaks in such a way that there was no added risk and stress because a nurse is on her break?

Actually, there is a "new technology" that is seeing impressive success in business.[22] Nurses are experienced leaders in its use and application. The "technology of care" may sound mushy to some, but it is a soft skill that expresses through your decisions, actions and the way you do something.[23] While it doesn't have to take extra time, it requires presence and the energy of intention that is more efficiently cultivated in a healthy environment. There is a lot of positivity research which suggests that an environment of kindness, created and practiced daily by companies, will lead to a happier workplace and an improved bottom line. It is likely that investing in and providing for the well-being of nurses will lead to better health for nurses, patients, and communities. It is further likely that a health-promoting lifestyle will reduce stress and chronic disease. These should eventually lead to a less burdened healthcare system. I invite you, my colleagues, to lead the way by taking care of your own health, which no one can do for you. Have care for yourself so you can continue to care and let nothing impede the delivery of your care.

Environment influences health. A healthy environment is essential for health. From the ecosystem of the planet, to the energetics of our emotions, and the ecosystem that modern science is most recently acknowledging – the microbiome of our gut – environment matters.[24] There is much to learn in this realm of knowledge and likewise much to gain from integrating its wisdom due to the interdependence of all these environments.

It is more commonly known than practiced in mainstream medicine that "genetics loads the gun, environment pulls the trigger," according to Dr. Francis Collins, director of the National Institutes of Health (NIH).[25] Stem cell research in the nineteen sixties by Dr Bruce Lipton's research proved that stem cell differentiation was influenced by the medium (environment) that the cells were put into.[26] This is a big reason that environment is so important and foundational to gene expression. You are less a victim of your genes than conventionally presumed.

🐑 This is a simple purging activity to allow you to express anything you need to before going on, similar to the pre-paratory stress dump in the Introduction. In your journal, write anything that is coming up for you – to set it aside, out of the way. So far, there has been a lot of information revealed from myself and you. How is it going? How are you doing? What is stirring, burning, fracturing or gell-ing in you? Lay it down on the page. Note what you find challenging, what issues come to light and any thoughts, conversations or actions that arise. This will move out any-thing cluttering your mind, giving it a place so that you do not have to carry it with you. But it is there in your journal to refer to and reflect upon if you want.

Advancing your knowledge will facilitate shifting from the prevail-ing story of competition, scarcity and victim-hood. This is groundwork for healing.

CHAPTER 4

STRESS AND HEALING

We have looked at how stress is prominent in our culture and seems integral to your job. Hopefully, you accept that you are not alone amongst your colleagues. Though peer and job pressures may imply otherwise, to admit you're feeling stressed takes courage and does not mean you are a less capable nurse, It is not your fault, and most important, despite feeling drained or powerless, you can do things to answer your inner call light. You must do this for yourself, because living in stress or fear doesn't support vitality and health.

A wise man was asked what surprises him the most, he offered this insightful response: "Man. Because he sacrifices his health in order to make money. Then he sacrifices money to recuperate his health. And then he is so anxious about the future that he does not enjoy the present; the result being that he does not live in the present or the future. He lives as if he is never going to die, and then dies having never really lived.[1]

Refer to the list you made in your journal of stressors you experience. Circle any you would credit to your job or workplace. For clarity, copy these to another page and you can add to the list. You can also combine the background stressors from Chapter 3 if they are a concern for you. You will interact with these in upcoming activities.

The Four Types of Stress

In his book, *Stress and the Manager*, Dr. Karl Albrecht, a pioneer in stress reduction training for business people, defined four common types of stress. They are time, anticipatory, situational and encounter stress.[2] Let's explore each of these.

Time Stress

If anyone knows this stress, you do. There is never enough time, whether on the job or a day off. Common ways to handle time stress address the managemental of time. To start earlier or stay later is not usually an option for nurses because of stringency around overtime. The natural tendency to cut corners is not a sustainable solution. Think back to Lucy and Ethel at the candy factory assembly line mentioned in the Preface. Cutting corners can make it look as if the work is done, but usually at a price. In your job, cutting corners could slight a patient, be a break in policy or practice, or otherwise be severely detrimental.

Have you endured any of the time studies done at work? These involve tracking everything you do your entire shift. Usually you document the time you enter and leave a specified area, when you start and stop a procedure, and every other activity during your day. Evaluating use of time, how it's delayed and where it's lost can improve efficiency, help with work flow, streamline methods and practices, and ultimately businesses hope it will improve cost effectiveness and processes.

Time is a potent stressor for you as a nurse. It is a commodity in the business of your work. The competition for your time is between the tasks and the patient; your self-care ought to be somewhere in the equation, too. According to a survey of Massachusetts nurses conducted by Anderson Robbins Research in 2018, "90 percent of nurses admit they lack adequate time to comfort and assist patients."[3] An article, "Ten Ways to Increase Nurses' Time at the Bedside" on *HealthLeadersMedia.com*, makes suggestions including those relating to bedside rounds, reporting and documentation along with other activities done at the bedside.[4]

This is not what you and your patients are likely talking about when referring to "time with the patient or nurse." Streamlining human interaction can be uncomfortable for you since you are the patient's interface or as I say, "the conduit of care."

You may have noticed that multitasking has not been mentioned. Recent studies show, "Multitasking is no longer a skill to brag about, but to worry about. These studies suggest multitasking causes us to make… more mistakes, retain less information, and change[s] the way our brain works…make us less productive…lowers IQ, decreases efficiency [and when] with a group of coworkers [it] creates a higher chance of miscommunication, missed deadlines, and poor work quality."[5]

Making a 'To-Do list' is a helpful way to organize tasks. Further prioritizing the list helps you focus on the more important tasks first, but does not assure that what is on the list will get done. The truth is lists get longer and nurses juggle tasks, constantly re-prioritizing and sometimes delegating. Clear face-to-face communication will facilitate group quality and efficiency of work.

Go back to your list of job stressors and put "T" beside the ones that are time related.

Anticipatory Stress

Associated with a coming situation or event that may or may not occur, this stress can cause a feeling of dread, angst, or anxiety. It can start the night before your shift, or while awaiting an admission to the room where the prior patient died. It can occur when the phone rings in the early morning of a day off or when on-call. The 'not knowing if or when' you could have to report for duty interferes with enjoyment or usage of your time. You may have difficultly focusing on your children's homework, relaxing with the family for movie night or getting to sleep.

Ways to curb anticipatory stress include being honest with yourself about your fears or insecurities and having a contingency plan in case something derails or changes. Clarifying what you truly dislike, dread or are afraid of will help put things into a more workable perspective. It can simplify the drama when you see things as they are for you and discover where to aim your efforts for resolution. When you expect something you dread, you are visualizing and focusing on the negative or undesired circumstances. Energy flows into the focus of your attention. Meditation can help ease your mind, calm the anxiety related to anticipatory stress and help you *shift* your focus to what you desire. Once you are honest with yourself and name the issue, you can choose to see it in a positive visualization that you intentionally create. With that resulting picture in mind, you have set an influential intention or tone from which to move forward.

(®) Go back to your list of job stressors and put "A" beside the ones that are anticipation related.

Situational Stress

It is common for people to experience surprises as stressful. Situational stress is circumstantial, such as in an emergency, getting called into your manager's office, feeling rushed or using a new piece of equipment. These are unanticipated situations in which you have less control. They may be incidental or they may resemble a prior situation or pattern in your life. In this case, it may magnify your stress because you respond from the mindset or emotion of the prior situation it resembles. Either way, you can feel powerless and unsupported. Becoming more self-aware and managing your emotions through learning to ground, center, and be present are ways to deal with situational stress that are explored in the AH SUCCESS Process. Also, learning communication skills and conflict resolution may be helpful.

(®) Go back to your list of job stressors and put "S" beside the ones that are situation related.

Encounter Stress

Encounter stress centers on people. People skills are necessary for personal interactions, especially when *you or they* are in distress as with patients, family members, colleagues, and even managers. Using self-awareness to get to know your emotions will help you recognize and understand them in others. Along with knowing yourself deeply, other nurse-survival tools are having empathy and using breathing techniques.

(♻) Go back to your list of job stressors and put "E" beside the ones that are encounter related.

Have you ever tried meditation, visualization, or relaxation techniques? What was it like for you? What was challenging? What was successful? Where do you see that any of these could be a helpful skill to have for your job, particularly related to each of these four types of stress? List these in your journal for recall and implementation. Also, make notes of encouragement. Learn from each time you encounter stress and intervene using one of your ideas.

The situation in this story about Jeanine and her stress might be familiar to you.

> Jeanine, a telephonic case manager, explained that she has 20 minutes to talk to each patient and 10 minutes to chart, then on to the next case. If something unexpected occurs, it is a delay in her work flow that can easily snowball her day and she will have to address them with her manager. She developed some compensatory steps to prepare for the shift and skillful techniques that achieve good results for handling time stress. Before she makes calls, she opens all the Electronic Health Record (EHR) charts. Then in each chart she pre-populates the shift note template for documenting the call. When talking with patients, she tells them the purpose of the call and their time allotment. Being respectful but assertive, she gives clear boundaries or choices to the patient rather than asking open-ended questions. This keeps the flow on pace for timely completion. She asks, for example, "Which choice do you want to make: change your diet to reduce your blood sugars or continue like you are with high blood sugars and not take part in this program?" Often she eats her lunch at her desk to allow time to send out communications to all necessary parties based upon the phone visit.

Do you recognize the stress Jeanine deals with and the coping mechanisms she uses to prepare, stay on schedule, and to catch up, thereby avoiding a meeting with her manager about productivity issues? Cutting marginally safe corners and pre-charting are things that streamline her required tasks and help her make it look like the tight time schedule works. She is accountable for her time, accuracy and compassionate care, and must achieve these defined metrics of success for the sake of her job.

While being respectful, Jeanine manages her time stress by using assertiveness with her patients to set the boundaries, provide choices and a review of accountability. This builds relationships with her patients based upon trust and empowerment. They like her because they know that she is straight with them and they can be honest with her.

Assertiveness training was the first continuing education (CE) class I attended. I asked to go instead of a clinical experience while in nursing school. The agreement with my instructor was that I do a seminar for my classmates about what I learned. This became my first educational program. In the early 1980s, when I took that class, nurses were working through the challenges of the slowly evolving nurse-doctor relationship. Most of the time, we no longer stood up to give our chair to a doctor, and we were speaking up if they were condescending to us. That seems crazy, doesn't it? Being assertive may seem difficult or uncomfortable to do, but this is not a means of confrontation. Rather, it is a means of communication. Assertiveness is standing up for yourself in a way that is sincere, direct and non-aggressive. In a non-emotional manner, you are stating what is true for you, using 'I-statements'. You remain calm, open and respectful.

Where could assertiveness be a helpful skill for you to use in your job, particularly related to each type of stress?

Stress, Inflammation and Health

Multiple sources link chronic stress to the six leading causes of death: heart disease, cancer, lung ailments, accidents, cirrhosis of the liver and suicide.[6] Over 75 percent of all physician office visits are for stress-related ailments and complaints.[7]

Below are some common effects of chronic stress in the body:[8,9]

- diminished cognition
- suppression of thyroid function
- blood sugar imbalances
- hormone dysregulation
- digestion maladies
- decreased bone density and muscle tissue
- tension
- increase in pain and the perception of pain
- raised blood pressure
- reduced immunity
- reduced ability to heal
- elevated "bad" cholesterol
- increased fat deposits around your abdomen
- increased risk for heart attack and stroke

Underlying these conditions is an inflamed internal milieu in the body. In the short term, inflammation is part of the healing process, whether a protective immune response to rid the body of a foreign invader, or to repair a broken or wounded part of the body.[10] Just like stress, when inflammation becomes chronic, it is damaging to our immune system and body. The ongoing presence of the stress hormone cortisol and pro-inflammatory cytokines in the body drive chronic low level inflammation. This contributes to an environment where 'the germ' can flourish and gene expression can switch on adaptively.[11, 12]

When stress becomes the norm, as it threatens to be for many nurses, it undermines health – especially from the dysregulation of the nervous and immune systems. It burdens an otherwise healthy system as it requires immense energy and depletes reserves of critical hormones and minerals causing damage to cells and tissues. Stress sabotages your best of intentions and relationships by diminishing mental focus and tolerance. A remarkable thing, revealed by working with many people on taming their stress, is that everyone experiences it differently.

There is much to learn from both the similarities and differences of their experiences. Common experiences of stress create changes in how the body functions, including emotions and personality. These changes are signals of the stress-related imbalance. Examples of potential changes can include:

- appetite
- digestion
- energy level
- motivation
- socialization
- tolerance

- breathing
- heart rate
- mood
- concentration
- muscle tension
- posture and gestures

The experience of stress can have a component of resistance because of a conflict of values, or a disparity in expectations or ability. Doing something that you are not in resonance with is taxing to your body. Overriding the internal signals, such as a strain in your gut, is confusing to body systems that are interdependent. A compensatory milieu may develop, perhaps leading to a symptom such as constipation or acid reflux. If you want to *shift* from stress to success, you will need to identify where your stress comes from, and get to know how you experience and react to it. Then you can learn to intervene, regulate your response to it and choose a course of action to resolve the cause. This is disarming the grip stress has on you and moving toward integrity with yourself. By this I mean cultivating honesty and respect between your conscience, brain, physiology, body, and heart.

Do what you know is right, ask for what you need and follow through on what you need to do – be it change your attitude or change your job. There is a continuum for stress. If it doesn't hurt you, your perception of it might. Often looking inward rather than outward for answers and resolutions will lead to the greatest success.

The meanings and associations you have with concepts and words are clues to unwinding the confusion you may have around why you are so stressed and possibly ill. It is important to consider your definition of some key concepts related to your health because these hold clues to both what constrains you and what you want. Ultimately, this affects what you create and the resulting experience.

(symbol) Make notes in your journal as you consider:
- » How do you define health? Illness? Well-being? Stress? Disease? Health care? Cure? Healing?
- » How are you influenced by the opinions of others?
- » Which is more important to you, autonomy or safety?
- » In any situation, would you rather be right or happy?
- » Which is better, quality or quantity?
- » Do you consider yourself healthy?
- » What attributes contribute to your view(s)?

Record your initial responses to:
- » For me, work is...
- » At work, I find it frustrating when...
- » Sometimes I feel _____ when _____.
- » I notice that I _____ when _____.
- » The thing that gets me the most about my job is...
- » On the job, I want to be _____.
- » If the pace at work is slow, I feel...
- » The pace at work is _____ and causes me to feel

  _____.
- » My time with my patients is _____ and makes me feel _____.
- » For me, time is _____.

Your answers to these exploratory questions are yours alone. They contribute to your world-view, experience of stressors and your picture of health. Write a description of your picture of health for yourself.

Autoimmunity, Stress and Environment

In the 1990s, they treated autoimmune illnesses as rare and isolated conditions. Autoimmune illnesses are seriously on the rise, thought to be from 50 to nearly 100 or more types.[13]

"Autoimmune illnesses are now [in 2011] recognized as among the leading causes of death for young and middle-aged women in the United States," according to Fred Miller, Director of the Environmental Autoimmunity Group at the National Institute of Environmental Health Sciences.[14] He further explains, "Prevalence rates for some of these illnesses are rising for what must largely be environmental reasons… Our gene sequences aren't changing fast enough to account for the increases." Miller added, "Yet our environment is – we've got 80,000 chemicals approved for use in commerce, but we know very little about their immune effects. Our lifestyles are also different than they were a few decades ago, and we're eating more processed food." Should prevalence rates for heart disease and cancer continue their decline, Miller says, autoimmune diseases could become some of the costliest and most burdensome illnesses in the United States.[15]

How many of these chemicals are you exposed to? 'Approved for commerce' does not equate to supporting health in your body. If you are not proactive by limiting or preventing exposure, you limit your options to settling for early recognition of symptoms and hope for intervention.

Are you connecting the dots from this information? Both fight-or-flight and chronic stress are associated with sympathetic stimulation. The dominant hormones present during stress affect immune function. It is deleterious to organs and body systems to be bathed in this neurochemistry repeatedly and ongoing. These become a condition of *dis-ease* and *ill-ness* on cellular levels, and the occurrence is on the rise because of environmental reasons.

Symptoms

Just over midway in my nursing career, I experienced symptoms that I eventually attributed to job stress, such as fatigue unrelieved by rest, brain fog and loss of satisfaction. I endeavored to maintain a positive attitude, get more rest, eat *right* and exercise, but I started gaining weight. I wondered what was going wrong with me.

I had a slim abdomen and pear-shaped body. I ate consciously and exercised regularly because I valued my health and fitness. I had followed a vegetarian diet with low to no dietary fat or added salt, like the prescription for cardiac patients. It surprised me when I noticed that I had developed a 'muffin top'. I was aware of its association with the stress hormone cortisol and metabolic disease. This made little sense with my lifestyle. There was no family history to support cardiovascular disease or diabetes. But it could make sense within the environment of my job.

Next, there was a six-week period where I was getting very little sleep each night. I initially reasoned that I was on adrenaline overload from the pace, acuities and lack of support on the job. I worked steadily through the day, not even thinking to take a break and would continue on into overtime as necessary. I would come home exhausted and crash on the couch, napping for hours and wrecking my chance of sleeping through the night. I knew this wasn't good, but my job came with productivity and stamina expectations.

Then followed several weeks of waking up at night with my clothes, and bedding soaked from sweating. You are wondering why I did not go to the doctor? Well, as a nurse, I had to figure out what is wrong so I could decide which doctor to call.[16] Serious things went through my head like menopause, TB and cancer.

Then one day at work a colleague asked if I was losing weight. I usually wore loose fitting scrubs, so I had not noticed that my scrub pants were more baggy. I attributed it to the fact I had two weeks off, which meant that I was not indulging in the delicious chocolates that were most always available, thanks to the thoughtful expression of appreciation from our patients. However, I continued to lose weight without trying despite an even more impressively insatiable appetite.

I sought the care of a Doctor of Osteopathy (DO). I had hoped to benefit from their nutritional knowledge and perhaps a broader perspective on treatment than a conventional Allopathic Doctor (Medical Doctor or MD) usually offered.[17] In the *two months before my appointment arrived*, I continued to lose weight, nearly 20 pounds total, and had made my self-diagnosis. The defining symptom was when I realized that my heart was beating hard and fast one day at work. I usually walked six to eight miles a day on my job, at a swift pace, but this felt different from an exercise-related increase in heart rate. It was bounding and persistent despite rest. The realization halted me, as I reached up to feel the enlarged outline of the thyroid gland in my neck. I knew the potential seriousness of this condition, hyperthyroid, and the standard medical treatments for it frightened me.

When the DO confirmed the diagnosis, she also confirmed the customary options for treatment. She had no other treatments or options to offer, which disappointed me, and the reality she painted deeply affected me. I felt pummeled by the experience of shock, denial, and bargaining as grief and fear rushed through me. She referred me for further diagnostic studies and to an endocrinologist. The endocrinologist concurred with the treatment plan from the DO.

The choices presented were: (a) Radioactive iodine; (b) A medication that destroys the thyroid and would likely also damage the liver; or (c) Surgical removal of the thyroid. I could not accept these as my only choices, so I chose (d) Find another option.

Personal Story as a Bridge Back to Health

Added to the job stress, I now had a serious situation of ill health for which the treatments were stress-inducing for me. I wondered how to get well and still handle the stress I was experiencing. No matter how this played out I would do anything I could to understand the symptoms, have them guide me to the root cause and re-balance my body, being and life. Professionally, I had also been in well-being and holistic practice since 1987, and it looked like this would be my chance to learn through my experience. There was nothing like a good dose of reality, such as the symptoms of a serious condition in my body, to wake me up. The focusing quality of the diagnosis provided a crystal clear perspective of things for me. I immediately could see, metaphorically, what such symptoms could mean and it made deep-sense. For me, having a diagnosis came with a big sense of *responsibility*. I seriously committed to my healing and used this opportunity to develop my *ability-to-respond* to life in healthier and more sustainable ways. I also had a feeling deep inside – deeper than the fear of the diagnosis and treatment – that I was going to be okay.

I did a holistic[18] assessment of myself, the symptoms, and my life, including my job, as if I was a client in my well-being practice. I had witnessed their courage to look deeply inward for answers and implement any wisdom they found. Despite the statistics and prognosis, I held the space for complete healing and had the intention to learn from the symptoms. I could not *see* myself doing A, B or C. But I *knew* deep inside my heart it was possible and within my ability to re-balance my life and symptoms. I visualized myself healthy and whole. Determined to walk the path of realizing health, food became my medicine. I also knew that I needed to improve my relationship with myself to be successful. I mindfully practiced until I successfully cultivated the feeling of a resilient, synchronized state of being in my mind, body and heart. Then I endeavored to maintain it, which required my ongoing intentional participation.

I found a Naturopathic Doctor (ND)[19] to work with and to guide the overall treatment plan. I am not suggesting any medical correlation of symptoms, diagnosis, or treatment, nor denying any. I am presenting this holistically[20] and revealing my perceived options. Any choices come with risks. I am not suggesting that anyone take the path I chose as it may not be for everyone, but it was the path for me. There are no guarantees for the outcomes in any treatment. Mainstream medicine reminds us of this each time we read disclaimers and sign consent forms.

I deeply committed to the rigorous necessary personal, dietary and lifestyle modifications to reduce anything irritating or inflammatory. Specific lab tests determined this and by following my Conscious Living Education™.[21] The latter is the program that had been the foundation of my well-being consultation practice since 1992. I used it to guide my self-assessment and modalities for self-regulation and care. As I studied the milieu of my life, I reviewed several recent major transitions in my life and, even more important, my reactions to them. I realized I had dismissed their relevance, but was seeing a deeper extent of their impact than was previously clear for me.

The impact of the more recent significant life change, moving state-side after living in the Caribbean, was easy to read in hindsight. Much of the change was beneficial, but stressful, and the components that challenged me were *very* challenging for me. I saw the origins of my stress and hence the "genetics" of the symptoms which exposed themselves in my area of metaphorical vulnerability – the throat. I had to 'swallow my feelings' to cope. I was trying to adapt to the state-side culture and healthcare environment which differed from the island community I had integrated into. This dominating disparity created a blockage of expression of my values, talents, creativity, knowledge and health. I had to moderate my interactions and reactions for my well-being because to be empowered I needed to act rather than react

Years prior, a friend worked in the Peace Corps for several years. When she returned to the States, she shared with me that it was easier to simplify and live the cultural values of the remote, impoverished village in Costa Rica than it was to reintegrate back in to the culture of the States. I now had a better understanding of what she meant and reflected on how the people of the Caribbean celebrated life compared to the the rush and competition in the States.

Metaphor and Healing

Metaphors are helpful for healing and understanding of symptoms. They are not physical or psychological but metaphysical, meaning above or beyond the physical. They are not literal, but more symbolic. Louise L. Hay provides a list of suggested metaphorical causes for symptoms in her book, *Heal Your Body: The Mental Causes for Physical Illness and the Metaphysical Way to Overcome Them.*[22] Looking further into my symptoms, with the help of Louise's book, a hyper-thyroid can be associated with humiliation and rage from being left out, lack of expressions or speaking one's truth. Wow, these are tough things to admit. But they shed the light of awareness on the places from where I could regain energy, power and health.

From my ND's perspective, I needed to detox from heavy metals, parasites and toxins. I needed to heal and cultivate a healthy intestinal microbiome, eliminate anything inflammatory and facilitate the easing of my overactive immune system, including stress reduction. For me, this was a stress-related, environmental and internal conflict induced illness that I was suffering and my ND embraced that perspective. Everything confirmed that I needed my personal integrity, power and health back, and I had lots of inner and outer work to do.

> Did you hear any of my values and personal definitions in my story? What environmental or lifestyle issues, or clues to my picture of health did you notice? How do you think any of those elements might contribute to disease, particularly autoimmune disorders? Review the story and note your elicited and related feelings, thoughts or ideas.

Life Changes and Stress

These words of Heraclitus, the pre-Socratic Greek philosopher, remain true today, "The only thing that is constant is change."[23] The natural tendency of the body is toward health and homeostasis. It's interesting that neither is a fixed state, but rather one of flux or change within counterbalancing parameters for vitality. An upset in this balance purposefully signals the body to adapt and re-establish homeostasis. These processes are ionic and chemical formulas for health and must be managed so as to not overwhelm the inherent resilience of body systems.

I had many life-changes in a condensed period prior to the occurrence of adrenal fatigue[24] and thyroid symptoms. The accumulation of changes took their toll on my health. Even though I knew the impact of stress on well-being, I did not realize at the time what was happening in my own life. This exemplifies that knowledge may be power, but *it's with the application of the knowledge that one becomes empowered.* It also highlights the importance of self awareness on many levels.

In 1967, The Journal of Psychosomatic Research published "The Social Readjustment Rating Scale," created by Thomas Holmes and

Richard Rahe at the University of Washington School of Medicine.[25] The scale, also known as The Life Change Index, looked at common stressors associated with life changes and attempted to measure their impact on health. It remains a useful stress impact assessment tool. In fact, related studies showed that the stress of life changes from a prior year affected the health of a person in the following year. The effects of stress can be cumulative and can be different between people, even in the same family.

Check in with yourself and rate your current stress level in your life on the familiar 0-10 scale, zero being nil and ten being severe. Next, do the Life Change Index. Please find the questionnaire in the supporting materials. ⓘ It will help you gather information for your awareness. Use the results optimistically to realize what you have been dealing with and to make adjustments if needed.

How did you react to your score on the Life Change Index? Were you already aware of this assessment or were you surprised by your results? How did the results compare to what you perceived? What did you learn from doing the assessment? Add any of these stressors to your list if not already included, and if they are still situations you want to work with?

Put a check beside the stressors listed in the questionnaire you experience specifically in relation to your work, including changes in health, sleep and finances. Pick one of the check-marked stressors and imagine yourself there now in an experience of the stressful thing. Engage all of your senses for information about your experience. Observe the scenario for several minutes (as long as you feel safe doing so) and make notes of realizations as they come.

» What is your facial expression? For instance, are your brows furrowed?

» What happens to your neck or shoulders, your breathing or posture?

» Any changes in your scalp, hands, jaw, stomach, buttocks, legs or feet?

» What are you learning about the way you experience stress at work or related to work?

» How does it affect your personality, emotions or interactions, for instance do you become impatient or quiet?

» Do you feel like taking any action or not?

Stop imagining that experience and let it go – the visualization, the feelings and thoughts.

Accept a deep, refreshing breath into your body. Exhale and sigh out loud with relief, and affirm you are here, now, safe and comfortable.

» How vividly did you experience the feeling of being stressed at work?

» Being honest with yourself, how stressed are you and how does stress affect you and your life? Your work?

» In what ways does it affect your ability to provide efficient patient care?

» How does it affect your ability to provide open-hearted care?

» What effects on your relationships with your nurse co-workers or manager can you attribute to stress?

» What effects on your personal life can you attribute to work stress?

If you could watch the scenario and feel it happening to you, you would more easily comprehend that your mind and body respond to imagined and remembered stimuli just as if it were actually occurring. Allow that concept to sink in. The neurochemical reactions are happening and the experience of their effects are the same with the 'perception' of something actual, imagined or remembered.

This phenomenon contributes to how we become reactive to situations and why people react differently. The effect of this is that the familiarity of a situation can stimulate a reaction without us thinking about it. Your brain responds under the powerful influence of your beliefs based upon prior experiences recorded into the subconscious. You automatically become defensive, dismissive, or trusting and relaxed by the power of your thoughts driving your autonomic nervous system. This suggests that much of your experience comes down to pre-cognitive perception, placebo, and as the Shuar suggested – the dream you hold.

Does this make it seem like your experience of stress is reactionary, out of your reach or beyond your control? New thought and emerging science reveal that through self-regulation techniques, such as the ones connected with the AH SUCCESS Process, can retrain the nervous system, brain and body.

Consider everything that falls onto your plate of responsibility and list as many in your journal as you wish. Marvel at everything you handle in your life. If you have *a story* – or when you become aware of *your story* – record it in your journal. As you saw with my symptoms and story, a personal story can contribute to understanding and help resolve illness. You are not stuck with your story and can, with intention, turn the page and write a new chapter in your story if you choose. You will learn in Part Two how to move beyond your stress to health and empowerment.

Nurses Do Stress With a Smile

When people in a social situation learn that you are a nurse, how do they respond? The most common answer recounted to me is one of warm and fuzzy gratitude. Next they may acknowledge it is hard and stressful work and say they could never do it. Most lay-people (and maybe some managers and executives) cannot comprehend the complexity and the breadth of the demands in your job.

There are emergencies you face when caring for people who are ill. Also, tender moments of intimacy, and relationships that you become involved in for little bits of time, only to lose them by a change in health or work assignment. These challenges require your nimble success at dealing with them on the spot, sensitively, intelligently and professionally. While that may be the normal fabric of the job of a nurse, please credit yourself for having the emotional, physical and mental capacity to carry on. In modern healthcare, there is a distinct struggle with increased intensity and complexity. Nurses must bear the modern unrelenting pressures of time and intensity by maintaining an additional basic underlying alert readiness. This is part of the increasing chronic low level of stress that burns and feeds dysregulated inflammation.

It takes courage to admit that you are experiencing job stress. The display of courage is an emotional-energetic threshold for personal growth and human potential, according to the "Scale of Consciousness". Developed from his research, Dr. David R. Hawkins, MD PhD, reveals that "displaying courage is achieved through a profound shift from destructive and life depleting behavior to life-promoting behavior and an integrity-based lifestyle."[26] Will you grant yourself this power over your stress by virtue of your courage to seek knowledge to help answer your inner call light?

As the Nurse's Stress Survey shows, your colleagues are realizing this for themselves. Courage is rising within nurses. It is empowering for nurses to speak up and to gain the ability to influence in this way. Most of the world is operating on the levels of fear and illness according to Dr. Hawkins' research. When you show courage from the heart for the sake of good and health, you are a counterbalancing force to the effects of those who are not.

Maybe nurses smile through the stress because it is an instinct to give a smile to someone is without one, such as a patient. There is something special about your smiling face beyond being good for customer service. Its true value is that it stimulates healing.

Smiling changes your physiology from stress to ease, powering up your capacity for healing. A radiant smile results from the vibratory synchrony throughout your body and being.

When someone is in pain or waking from anesthesia, your smile warms and reassures them, even when you just grin to bear it. Research shows that when you smile or just turn up the corners of your mouth, it reduces your stress and is good for your heart.[27]

(☺) Be seated and take notice how you feel. Close your eyes, then smile and notice how you feel differently. Feel the smile on your face. Feel it in your mind. Feel the smile in your neck and shoulders. Smile with your heart... and your liver... and down to your toes. Radiate the feeling of your smile throughout your body. How do you feel? Alternate smiling and not smiling, the corners of your mouth up and down. Notice the shifts? Describe the feeling of these shifts and summarize your experience in your journal.

Practice noticing how you feel and whether you are smiling throughout your day. Feel the shift as you smile and feel your well-being. When you beam from the inside out, a patient will feel it. So keep smiling because it increases your face value and reduces the negative effects of stress for yourself and your patients.

Adaptation and Stress

Dr. Hans Selye, a Hungarian-Canadian Endocrinologist, known as The Father of Stress, introduced The General Adaptation Syndrome (GAS).[28] This syndrome introduced a stress response model of how Dr. Selye described moving through the phases of stress. Alarm is characteristic of the acute phase. This involves protective mechanisms that are imperative for immediate survival and self-preservation. If stress continues, the body progresses into resistance where it must accommodate the ongoing demands or strains. This is not a sustainable state, as personal resources become gradually depleted. During either of these first two stages, physiological and cellular recovery can occur when the threat has ceased and the body re-balances.

In humor you may think alarm and resistance are a part of most any day at work for you. You may even feel you thrive on stress, because of the concept of hormesis where a little stress builds stamina or what doesn't kill you will make you stronger. But seriously, even while there is eustress, positive stress that has positive effects on the body, if the stress remains unresolved, and continues for an extended period, depletion, damage and exhaustion will result.

Research has lead to new understanding of the cellular health and the important role of mitochondria – the energy generators inside each cell – in health, chronic illness and aging. The long term effects of depletion include cell destruction, immune system failure, body system malfunction and even death.[29] Imagine the cascade of issues that must have occurred within my body that showed up as an auto-immune thyroid condition. Severe chronic stress depleted the regulatory systems of my body to the point of developing unhealthy or malfunctioning thyroid cells, which were attacked and potentially destroyed by my immune system because they weren't acting right. My immune system was doing what it is supposed to do, except it stopped recognizing the cells as 'self'!

Let's look at models that suggest how degradation into ill-health may happen.

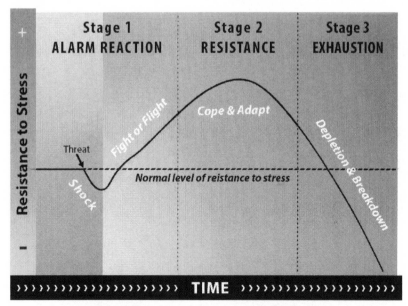

Dr. Hans Selye's General Adaptation Syndrome (GAS)
Graphic adapted by Vivo Digital Arts

There are many perspectives on health and illness that correlate with the GAS model of progressive system imbalance leading to disease or system failure and suggesting that reversal of the dysregulation is feasible up to a point.[30] ⓘ The following are brief summaries of several such models.

- Emotionally: There are two basic states – love and fear. The physiology of Love is dominated by life enhancing hormones which create an internal environment for happiness, health and healing to occur. Stress hormones dominate the physiology of fear, as in the resistance and exhaustion stages of GAS.

- Physiologically, there are two states. The state of ease which supports health and healing, and the state of dis-ease, which literally means difficult or without ease. Dis-ease is a degrading condition exhibiting acute to chronic symptoms, often with debilitating and terminal circumstances.

- The Electromagnetic perspective uses intelligent energy management as developed by Dr. Childre and the researchers at HeartMath Institute. There is a spectrum of states involving emotions and energy (or level of stimulation) that span from Depletion to Renewal.[31] These concepts are a way of understanding the interplay of emotions, hormones and nervous system during stress, recovery and building resilience through coherence using the science of heart rate variability and electromagnetics.

- A bioregulatory systems approach appreciates the patients' autoregulatory capacity. It relates disease complexity to an individual's homeostatic systems and their interactions across all levels of biological organization.[32]

- Homotoxicology is based upon effects of toxins on the body, and illness often depends on the intensity and duration of toxic blockages and the body's natural ability to detoxify or eliminate such threatening poisons. There are four stages of disease from acute to degenerative.[33]

- Immunologically there are the two states, over- or underactive, which lead to autoimmune breakdown or over growth abnormalities, respectively.[34]

- Metabolically, the breakdown, elimination, detoxification and repair processes of the body are in balance and efficient in optimal states. Under the effects of stress hormones, imbalances occur that lead to dysregulation, breakdown and disease.

- Cellularly, the body operates in the chemistry of safety or danger resulting from the signaling from multiple levels of surveilling systems, such as emotional, chemical, immunological, and neurological. The cutting-edge research by Robert Naviaux, MD PhD, in Mitochondria Medicine holds that the mitochondria, known as the powerhouse of a cell for manufacturing energy, is integral to the healing state of the body via sensing how to regulate the flow of energy – into health maintenance or survival in response to chemical, physical, microbial. or emotional threats. These two different forms of metabolism that cannot concurrently exist and contribute to the experience of vitality or fatigue.[35]

- Environmentally, health is about diversity, cooperation and balance. A natural environment with sustainable use and cultivation of resources is life and health enhancing. The quality of our inner nature (health) declines within a resource depleted and toxic external environment because of their interdependence.

Do any of these perspectives make it plausible for you that physiological imbalances such as with stress can contribute to disease and illness? Does any of this information validate why you experience the effects of your stress so deeply, even in your cells, as insatiable fatigue, or an alarming inner call light? Consider the potential role of stress in adrenal fatigue, inflammatory and autoimmune thyroid symptoms, or a symptom that you may be experiencing. Journal about your ideas, hunches and realizations about the relationship between your experience of stress and health.

Amygdala Hijack

Meet Rachel, a labor and delivery (L&D) nurse, faced with stress, challenge and competition in her young career.

Rachel briskly walked into the L&D (labor and delivery unit) nurses' station, reached for coffee and claimed her place at the desk in nearly a single well-practiced movement.

Women were on gurneys, laboring in the hallways – it was already a busy day.

Her heart was already beating fast – initially jump-started by the urgent phone plea that morning, to come in to work on her day off – she felt the jolt of the caffeine perking up her sleep-deprived brain and clearing her bleary early morning vision. The manager breezed through the station. "You're in postpartum, Rachel."

Rachel immediately snapped and stiffened her posture.

"What? Why? I always work in L&D." *Have I done something wrong? Am I losing rank? Why is my manager questioning my ability? I'm a high achiever and cool under pressure kind of nurse. My talents belong in L&D. Why am I being assigned to work the "snooze fest" on postpartum?*

Despite her questions, the manager restated the assignment.

Rachel stood, turned on her heels, walked through the nursery and out the nearest exit, slamming the door behind.

A moment later, Rachel sheepishly re-entered the nursery through the same door.

Thank goodness for the building codes that required shatter-proof glass in doors to protect innocent infants from sleep deprived, over-worked, competitive, adrenaline driven, scared-we-are-not-good-enough, new nurses under mounting job pressures, like me.

She knew the instant that the door left her hand, that she was making a huge mistake.

What just happened?

Rachel's mind cleared as she realized her exhaustion and felt the entity that commandeered her brain and body slowly withdraw itself. With the risk of her actions being documented as insubordinate, the only thing she could do was admit that she reacted inappropriately while professing she would improve her attitude and do her assignment.

In short-term stress, it may be easier to identify the source, eliminate it or get to safety and recover. This is stimulating and challenging to the body, but easy to recover from. It seems to be a common experience with chronic stress to have the feeling of being chased or not being able to get caught up, as if on an endless treadmill.

With chronic stress, identifying the source can be more difficult because it is often a circumstance or a blend of things. It could be a general feeling or interpretation of a stressor that has become a habitual state of being or mood. It could also be a rapid succession of multiple stressors or events without recovery time that lead to overwhelming state and depletion of the body. The problem is that in modern society, including nurses' work environments, the stress mechanisms work repetitively and frequently, shunting energy and resources for survival and away from health maintenance and higher cognitive functioning.

Sometimes in fight-or-flight activation, a contextual trigger awakens a deep emotional memory, which can lead to a sudden, overwhelming, unconscious and seemingly disproportionate emotional response. This is an "amygdala hijack," coined by Daniel Goleman in his book Emotional Intelligence.[36]

Have you ever yelled at someone and then regretted it later, realizing that you overreacted? Have you been upset while in traffic or while waiting in a store check-out line? How about while having to wait for the delivery of a medication from pharmacy amidst your shift that is snowballing? Any "yes" means you have been a victim of an amygdala hijack.

You have likely seen this occur involving patients and family members in crowded waiting rooms where fear and emotions run high. Or maybe a patient who felt your response time was too slow to their request for pain medication, unloaded their feelings onto you. This happens because the emotional brain responds for survival before the thinking brain can reason. When the thinking brain catches up, the area and people around you are already scorched. You may feel remorse, even fatigue, but likely do not know what just happened.

Describe the setup for an incident that led to a time when you overreacted. What was your state (physical, emotional, etc.) and how did you feel before and after? Describe your reaction.

What triggered your reaction? What excuse did you use or blame for any outburst you might have had? Could you recognize a similar reaction occurring within you in another situation? How would you know? How would you intervene or handle it differently? Note your answers in your journal for further contemplation.

The circumstances of an episode like this are usually complex, and many variables are not within your control. An amygdala hijack is a severe symptom. Systems, practices and relationships need review for intervention. But keeping this about you and your well-being, you must direct self-care at these levels, ideally at the moment and ongoing. If you become depleted from ongoing stress and feelings of dis-empowerment the degradation of your internal neuro-chemical state and nervous system will undermine your abilities. Before this worsens or becomes chronic, you may need to seek nutritional, medical, counselor and employee (human resources, employee help line, labor union) support.

> ♥ If you are feeling residual discomfort from recalling that experience, you can ease it quickly by visualizing the person or group and saying, "I apologize for my behavior. Thank you for accepting my apology." Then let yourself earnestly know that you will do better next time. Exhale and feel the relief. Then breathe in optimism and self-trust. Spend a few moments with this to recover.

The good news is that you can learn to recognize the onset of this in yourself and others, and learn to get out of the way, intervene and recover from it. You can keep your center of higher reasoning in the prefrontal cortex of your brain operational and discerning if you manage it. This is beneficial to be skilled at doing because effects from the flood of epinephrine (adrenaline) and cortisol, that may be unnecessary and excessive, can remain in your system for several hours after an incident of activation. Your body systems will remain hyper-stimulated until they steadily cool down and recover. How many times do you get activated in a day at work? Learning to control your response – both outward bursts and inward seething stoicism – and calm down more quickly is healthy, empowering, and will lead to far better outcomes.

Think of your patients. They are likely in a stress-response condition with their diagnosis, treatments and concerns. Your calm, centered and knowledgeable presence is necessary as a refreshment and stabilizer for them. Because only one side of the autonomic nervous system can be stimulated at a time, they will resonate with your calm presence and shift out of fear to relaxation. They cannot concurrently experience fear and relaxation, or heal while under the influence of stress hormones. Both you and your patients will benefit from your self-care and ability to self-regulate your emotions, attitudes and stress response. Your patients will benefit even more if you teach them how to shift from stress to relaxation to heal and build resiliency.

Relaxation and Resilience

Dr. Herbert Benson, professor, author, cardiologist, and founder of Harvard's Mind/Body Medical Institute, coined the term, *"Relaxation Response"*, which is also the title of his book.[37] The relaxation response is the antithesis of the stress response. By stimulating the parasympathetic nervous system you can counteract the physiological effects of stress. He showed the powerful effects of meditation to accomplish this. According to Marilyn Mitchell, MD, "Benson can be largely credited for demystifying meditation and helping to bring it into the mainstream." It is important to note that relaxation and resilience are not the same. Lack of this understanding can lead to misconceptions about relaxation and self-regulation techniques, their use, and effectiveness. Relaxation implies a slowing down. You need relaxation to counterbalance your stress and promote health. Obviously, you cannot stop and fully relax amidst an emergency because you must continue to function effectively. But you can self-regulate while continuing to function or downshift using the relaxation mechanisms, then spring back. This missing delineation is one reason people will say they do not have time for self-care or that the techniques are merely diversions.

While you can start immediately intervening with your stress and doing self-regulation, you find that practicing and efficient skill building can take time, attention and intention to master. This is because it does not come from knowing the information, but applying it effectively. Also, you are learning to augment, if not override, a potent automatic physiological reaction. Do not underrate relaxation, it is necessary for health and is part of the Yin-Yang balance of nature. But there are skills to use while in action to temper your stress response and maintain or improve your cognitive and physical abilities.

For this resilience, you must build knowledge and awareness about the different states of being and how you experience relaxation and stress. Resilience is a healthy state of physical and emotional elasticity, being able to bounce back with plenty of resources in reserve. The reserve is critical because chronic disrupted sleep, a nutrient-poor diet, and chronic stress deplete it. Cognitive understanding of the circumstances and learning to respond intelligently, which includes managing your energy and things that drain it, is what self-regulation can encompass for you. So practice in calm, safe and supportive environments, where you can deeply relax and rebuild your reserves. This way you learn how to sense the state of your reserves and the desired state to *shift* to when you recognize yourself being controlled by your overstimulated neurochemistry and emotions. Getting to know how you experience relaxation is important before you need to self-regulate during a code or amygdala hijack.

The Easy as A-B-C Technique

This is a useful self-regulation method I devised to help intervene when experiencing stress, such as the types we reviewed above. In 1991, when I worked in an emergency room, I began teaching the technique to patients and co-workers who found it helpful and effective for themselves. The emergency medical technicians (EMTs) also used it with the patients during ambulance transports. I crafted the *Easy as A-B-C Technique* based upon my experience with a diverse collection of skills and modalities. I found awareness, breathing and centering to be common, accessible and effective skills. The "A-B-Cs" is easy to remember and use on-the-spot when feeling stressed.

A is for Awareness:

Become aware of your experience.
Awareness responds to the
movement of your Breath.

B is for Breath:

Use your breath as the tool to
self-regulate. *Breath* is a guide that
is always available and is a potent
regulator of your nervous system.

C is for Center:

Then *shift* to your *Center*. Your
Center is a still space within
you that anchors and magnifies
awareness. This is the *place* to either
rest or respond from.

Check in with yourself and notice how you are doing and
feeling now. Do the A-B-Cs with the skill you have, even
if you don't think you have any. Do what comes to you.
Check in with yourself again. Notice and write any observations in your journal.

These are three important concepts that are also integral
to the AH SUCCESS Process and will be explored in more
detail in Part Two. You my discover a familiarity with these
intuitive concepts and be surprised at what you don't know
you know.

In the mid-1990s, while I was working with the Omega Institute, I learned validating science and history from the faculty which helped me further understand and trust the *Easy as A-B-C Technique*. I was fortunate to hear 'The Father of Mindfulness', Jon Kabat-Zinn, PhD, teach about mindfulness-based stress reduction which he first introduced in 1979. He co-pioneered the Stress Reduction Clinic at the University of Massachusetts Medical School, which developed into the Center for Mindfulness in Medicine, Health Care and Society. They use mindfulness for stress reduction, eating disorders, depression and much more.

Another faculty member of Omega, Daniel Goleman, PhD, an internationally known psychologist and author, spoke about Emotional Intelligence (EI), which he subsequently popularized in 1996. EI is about cultivating the ability to recognize, understand and manage emotions for yourself and others, especially when under pressure. This is a skill that will help you improve your experience of work, health and as you evolve as a leader. Amidst the ranks with your nurse-colleagues, cultivating emotional intelligence can reduce hostility and the experience of stress while team building and facilitating communication.

Faculty member, Candace Pert, PhD, a neuroscientist and a professor of physiology and biophysics at the Georgetown University School of Medicine, also inspired me. Known as The Mother of Psychoneuroimmunology (PNI) and The Goddess of Neuroscience, she "proved the science behind the mind-body-energy connection" when she discovered the opiate receptor in the brain and later the endorphin receptors in the body during her graduate research at Johns Hopkins University in 1978. PNI is the study of the relationship and effects of mind and emotion with the nervous and immune systems and their effects on health.

Dr. Pert once commented, "We've all heard about psychosomatic illness, but have you heard about psychosomatic wellness? Since emotions run every system in the body, don't underestimate their power to treat and heal."[38] Her point may bring validation and understanding to the significance of the placebo effect.

It is empowering to think we can shift stress into success to maintain health by regulating our attitudes, thoughts, emotions and physiology. Do you see or feel that potential gain in power over your health and well-being? It is said the only thing you can control or change in life is your mind, reactions and attitudes. This differs from holding an emotion inside which may be tactful to do in the short term but undermines health over time. Changing an unhealthy emotion results in a chemical change in the body affecting the internal physiological messages that run your nervous, immune and cardiovascular systems. Doing this will help you control the drain of your energy and, along with a nutrient-rich diet and healthy movement, can rebuild your depleted reserves to maintain and rebuild health. ⓘ

CHAPTER 5

WISDOM FROM STRESS

The difference between the tension (stress) and relaxation (being) according to a Chinese proverb is a matter of acceptance. Tension is who you think you should be and relaxation is who you are. Acceptance is a challenging thing to achieve in a culture that promotes striving, competing and winning. It may be a riddle worth contemplating why nature is cooperative, yet people compete. Research shows that plants are less caught up in an evolutionary struggle for survival than conventionally thought. They live in cooperation and share resources when crowded together, even making intentional effort to help one another.[1,2]

Relating back to our discussion on Maslow's pyramid in Chapter 3, what are we competing for and to what means? Will we ever be able to close this stress-related acceptance gap referred to in the Chinese proverb above? How can a person reach self-actualization at the tippy-top of Maslow's pyramid, which surely must involve acceptance? Finding wisdom in what causes stress can help release it. It can lead to meaning, perhaps through a dynamic balance of understanding as in the principles of Yin-Yang. Through the AH SUCCESS Process in Part Two, you will unlock wisdom from *your* stress, over and above the general information in this chapter.

Survival or Success

Without a healthy stress response, we humans would not survive. Your body learns from encounters that evoke a healthy stress response. Your brain and immune system are intrinsically conditioned for early recognition of and rapid responsiveness to a threat. Dr. Selye said that anything, positive or negative, can be experienced as stressful, because the same neurochemical reactions take place in the brain and body. His point is that the ones interpretation becomes defining.[3] Deadlines, bills, job interviews, public speaking or even a meeting in the manager's office are often sources of stress but are not life threatening. Because of this, stress – to a point – can be perceived as good, and motivate you toward success. This relationship between performance and health with a degree or duration of arousal (stress) starts out as motivating, promoting growth and health up to a peak state. If it persists however, stress can become excessive and diminish performance and health over time. Note in the diagram below that fatigue is just over the crest of arousal from peak performance. This relationship was first described in 1908 by psychologists Robert Yerkes and John Dillingham Dodson, whose work is the basis of the graph.[4]

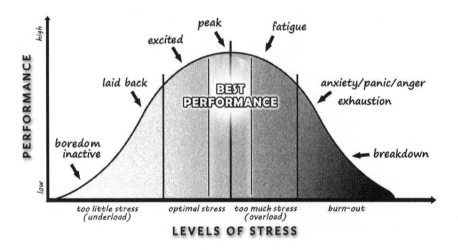

Influence of levels of stress on performance & wellbeing, based upon the Yerkes-Dodson Law.
Graph licensed from Adobe Stock / desdemona72 - adapted by Vivo Digital Arts

The primitive nerve cell firings that raise the alarm by releasing chemicals like adrenaline, noradrenaline and cortisol into the bloodstream affect your inner call light. You must learn to recognize how you are functioning and modulate effectively. The neurochemicals of stress range in effect from sharpening senses to stupefying. Motivation can turn into apathy, courage into fear, and passion into anger with chronic exposure to this stress environment.

Within Stress Lies Energy for Health

Energy tied up in the stress of anticipation, regret, coping and arguing fuels the fire of stress through fight-or-flight activation. This usurps energy from your well-being. It alters brain blood flow when under stress so mental confusion, including forgetfulness, is common during times of stress, even for professionals like nurses.[5]

Abraham Lincoln said, "When angry, count to ten. If very angry, count to one hundred."[6] This is good advice. During intense emotion the act of counting will restart the neocortex of your brain, which is shut down by the stress response, making it difficult to reason. By being present with the counting, you will experience some "distance" between yourself and the stress, reducing your potential emotional reactivity. Thus, your brain will operate in a much more energetically sustainable state. Your mind cannot remain simultaneously in stress and in relaxation; it has to *shift* and it naturally will when allowed. Handling stress effectively and addressing its causes will free energy for vital activities such as building health, relationships and happiness.

With Stress You Need No Other Enemy

We can liken ongoing stress to carrying a burden. The following Buddhist parable about carrying a burden and letting go shows this concept:

A senior Monk and a junior Monk were walking on a journey together. They came upon a lady crying because she needed to cross the river but felt she could not do it on her own.

The younger Monk hesitated. Without a word or gesture, the senior Monk picked her up and carried her across the river, set her down gently on the other side and continued on his way.

The younger Monk was shocked with disbelief of what he had observed.

When the younger Monk caught up with his companion, they walked in silence for a long while. The younger Monk was struggling with making sense of how the older Monk could so easily break his vow. The more he thought about it, the more upset and angry he became. As Monks, they could not touch a woman. Finally he asked the older Monk how he could do such a thing... break his vow and carry that woman. The older Monk asked, "What woman?" The younger Monk reminded him of the woman he carried across the river. The older Monk replied, "I set her down a long time ago, but you, my brother, are still carrying her."

Burdens have weight. Mental and emotional burdens can be experienced as a heaviness. Carrying extra weight for long periods of time is degrading to your body on all levels. The sensation of weight associated with a burden is due to the summation of the demand and resistance between mental, emotional, physical and energetic tensions.

The younger Monk, in the story above, strained over the incident far too long. He created the difficult journey for himself by working against himself. This is how stress seriously works against you and you need no other enemy because *you* are your own worse enemy. Often the biggest relief occurs when we finally let go of whatever burden we are carrying.

List things you carry such as stress, worry, blame, anticipation, guilt, even insecurity. Where or how do you feel their weight or burden? Write beside each burden how long ago it occurred or how long you have been carrying it. Also beside each, write any feeling associated with it. Are you willing to put down or let go of some of these things? What do you perceive it would take to put them down, let go? What's the flinch, angst, tug, pull, draw, resistance or hesitancy when you think about changing your relationship with that burden? Write your answers and prompts for further consideration.

Close your eyes and imagine peace between you and the other person, situation or thing, or trait within yourself. See the binding ties release. Feel space being created with room for new potential where there was the clutter of tangled old business. Watch that burden, that thing move further away until it is a speck that disappears. Notice your breath. How has it changed? Notice your brows, jaw, tongue, throat and shoulders. Any changes toward release and relaxation? Letting go is a freeing practice. Journal about anything that you learned about yourself, patterns of holding and willingness to let go. Describe the sensation of letting go and feeling relief.

Accept the slightest release as a success, a turning down of the volume. This is a process – learning how to de-stress, relax and release. Recognizing and owning your successful *shifts* will reinforce the accomplishment and help you be more likely to maintain it.

Creativity and The Release of Stress

One wisdom gleaned from experiencing unhealthy stress is that healing from it requires change. Creativity will facilitate healthy changes for stress relief. Author Joyce Carol Oates says, "Constant interruptions are the destruction of the imagination."[7] You must set aside the 'distraction free' time for yourself and your creativity – and keep it sacred. Engaging in creativity lifts you out of stress and into a world where anything is possible. Time warps, distractions vanish, and it transforms your neurochemistry into a healing state.

Apparently there is no neural network in the brain specifically responsible for creativity like there is for the modes of executive control, background scanning and prioritizing of what gets your attention. Dr. Brenner calls these the 'Big Three' brain networks, which according to research, appear to work together for creativity.[8] He says that "together they form a more comprehensive, responsive and resilient system which produces a neurological signature of creativity" that was identified and published by researchers Beaty and colleagues (2018).[9] The mode of creativity is one of growth, change and vitality.

Several years into my nursing career, I found a hobby. The joy of working in stained glass was amazing for me. Having a tangible creative outlet was a very healthy thing to engage with as a nurse with a stressful critical care job. The feat of perceiving something with my mind, achieving it with my hands and expressing originality through the process was thrilling.

Engaging in a creative outlet or hobby switches your mind, body and spirit into a different realm that can provide respite, boost your spirit or replenish your energy. I highly recommend that if you do not have a hobby or an expressive outlet that you seek one. It can be anything during which you can express yourself or that brings you joy – like karaoke singing, dancing, jogging, painting or playing guitar. Engaging in a hobby or expressive activity changes you because it requires a different neurochemistry and whole brain coordination.

In my first year as a working nurse, the poem, "Look Closer Nurse", was passed between nurses in the hospital. It was written by a nurse in Scotland, from the perspective of a "crabbit old woman" as a patient. She asks, "What do you see, nurse... when you're looking at me?" It is a call for her nurse to see the person, behind the dribbles, forgetfulness, helplessness and silence. [10,11]

What do you see when you look at a patient – a diagnosis, a treatment list, a complainer? That poem deeply touched me. I could hear the message, but wanted to defend parts and wanted a pardon for others. Emotion came from somewhere deep inside me in a poetic backlash of my squelched creativity. The irony was that through creativity I released my stress and emotions in a way of beauty.

I find poetry, even silly poetry, helps me let go of stress as my creativity flows. My "What Do You See, Patient?" poem was reflective and therapeutic. How do you relate?

What Do You See, Patient?

What do you see, patient,
what do you see?
What do you see
when you look at me?

A person who's never there
when you put on your light.
One who's distracted and busy,
can't get the IV right?

A person who is dumb
because the doctor said, *au
contraire.*
Someone disorganized
because so much is up in the
air?

I have three other patients,
they each need care too.
And then all I hear is,
"I called, Where were you?"

You wanted a pain pill
ten minutes ago.
I was in an emergency,
little did you know.

You called for some water,
but I didn't come stat,
I was cleaning an incontinence,
can you believe that?

At the moment you wanted
some ice in your pitcher,
I was mapping a rhythm
to check someone's ticker.

When you called for a straw,
I was feeding Ms. Sweet.
A dinner break for me?
No, I'll eat on my feet.

You think I'm one who cleans
bedpans,
handmaiden for a doc?
Well, I'll say to you, dear
patient,
"Just let me tell you what..."

I'm an individual, a student,
a mother, a wife.
I have responsibility while here,
and in my own life.

My car is broken,
I'm getting over the flu.
My bills aren't paid yet,
my mother is sick too.

My lover and I had
an argument, today,
All this I set aside
to serve you in this way.

Now that my shift is over
I still have paperwork to do.
You will think I'm long gone,
but I'll be here an hour or two.

After all work is done...
When did I last go pee?
For the past ten hours
I forgot about me!

— *Barbara Young RN, 1984*

🫀 What value does creativity hold for you? What merit does creativity hold in your job? In your journal write about what you do to be creative when you are not working. How does it help you? What have you learned about yourself from engaging in it? If you don't engage in a hobby or spend time in creativity, take a few moments to write what you would like to do. When might you find time to add creativity to your life?

Being creative can be actively taking part in a hobby or sport for enjoyment, or gardening, dancing, singing or anything else that is self-expressive. It is worth your effort to do so because cortisol (the stress hormone) reduces in saliva, after 45 minutes of engaging in a creative activity you enjoy.[12]

I remember being an adrenaline junkie during my career. The cutting edge of technology, the biting edge of making a decision when time was of essence, the fine line between life and death during a code... all yang expressions of energy, excitement and creativity. These job pressures were stimulating and engaged my interest. I also remember feeling that I had made a real difference during yin moments of stillness. Such a time was when a laboring patient told me that my holding counter-pressure on her sacrum to relieve her back labor helped her *shift* out of pain and into being present for the birth.

Some nurses report feeling their job has become like a treadmill that continues to speed up, leaving less time with their patients and no time for breaks. The pressure of the job not only reduces their satisfaction, but also their health because the body cannot rest or digest while humming on sympathetic physiology. Managers interested in time management and productivity may say they do not pay staff nurses to think creatively, but to just perform their job. A job like this resembles being on an assembly line. Unfortunately just following the achievement of proficiency, repetition can be disengaging. This in no way validates the abdication of your responsibilities, but it is important to understand if your position invites your creativity or not. Coloring inside the lines, so to speak, reduces stress of one kind, but may compound it for you otherwise. It may be challenging or impossible to find moments for creativity in your job or life. However, once you engage in creativity, life can be more meaningful.

There is balance to be found between the forces of job pressure and meaningfulness of work. Teresa Amabile, a professor at Harvard Business School, presents these concepts in her book, *The Progress Principle*. She contends that if at the end of the day your personal goals have not been engaged or met, the worth of putting up with the stress will be diminished and the job will be less meaningful.[13] This is unfortunately happening with nurses. If the measure of your accomplishments at the end of the day is based upon how many discharges and transfers you orchestrated, the number of medications you administered, how much faster you did a procedure and ultimately how much overtime pay you get in your next paycheck, then you should take note. Your performance review might be golden, but you will probably not feel satisfied in the long run and it may affect your health. Actively create your career to stay engaged and fulfil your satisfaction.

Stress can stimulate or suppress creativity. Some people say a deadline makes them get the job done. Others say that pressure to perform is inhibiting. Some people feel exhilarated by the bells and whistles of shiny technology, and others are de-energized by it. Some nurses crave time with their patients – ministering rather than just administering. It is important to consider how you become motivated, what your job creativity versus stress relationship is, and what balance you need to be healthy and happy.

The state of inspiration is a higher level of *being,* important for health and an antidote to stress. Creativity can bring you into a state of flow,[14] an experience of complete engagement in what you are doing and a lost sense of self, time, and space. You dissolve into the activity and the *do-ing* becomes *be-ing,* and it is intrinsically rewarding. This is a state of low resistance and high efficiency where thought expresses as form easily. Athletes commonly get into this flow as do artists, dancers, musicians and healers. They become the activity while doing it, and there is no wasted energy. Form is fluid, and every movement has both purpose and meaning. There's an inherent satisfaction in this way of *be-*

ing that satisfies more completely than your most favorite sweet, edible treat.

Do you get into a flow-state in your job as a nurse? I suggested earlier that you were likely a nurse at heart before going to school and getting a job. Then the job description defined what you do as a nurse. For you, how much disparity lies between being a nurse and doing the tasks of your job? Any disparity can contribute to your experience of job stress, while any congruence can help you gain momentum and lift out of the burden of your stress.

> Recall an experience of flow and answer these questions in your journal:
> » What were you doing? How were you *being*? What did you experience during the flow state? What was your breathing like?
> » What were you thinking? Were you thinking? What did you experience after re-emerging into awareness of time and your surroundings? What was the payoff for you?
> » How frequently do you experience this?

Imagine if you experienced flow in your life more often. When there is no experience of time pressure, there is no impedance to creativity. Your body and mind can be in dynamic ease. This unburdened state allows spontaneity and healing to occur, and becomes a state of sublime well-being. It is the natural tendency of the milieu within your body to seek balance and flow. Preventing external stress from impeding this internal flow and intentionally engaging in activities to enhance internal flow will help you balance the effects of stress. Creativity is nearly as important as sleeping well and eating for fuel and nutrition.

Paradigm Stress

A paradigm, is the body of beliefs, the usual way of thinking about or doing something, or the underlying assumptions held by an individual or a society.[15] While paradigms may be broad reaching in their application, it is difficult for them to encompass all aspects of cultures such as spiritual, financial, family, health and other factors that contribute to the whole of life. While a paradigm may become *the way*, it is only *a way*. Any disparity, when involved in several paradigms, can cause stress experienced as pressure, friction or a clash. This calls for balance and room for possibility to enter. We are looking in particular at the yin and yang of nursing and medicine in healthcare.

I had jobs as a waitress and a nurse-technician (nurse-tech) prior to my first job as a registered nurse. Waitressing provided excellent preparation and training for nursing by teaching necessary skills of customer service, handling complaints, rapport-building and organization, and working under pressure for efficiency and customer satisfaction. The nurse-tech position gave me a head start with channeling my desire to help people into specific skilled tasks, duties, treatments and policies for nursing. Both sets of skills were necessary, but the customer service skills have increased in value, particularly in the current times when "hospitals compete with one another... patients are customers... and lower costs, higher quality care and better patient outcomes [are commodities]."[16,17]

As a new nurse, I experienced a departure from the foundations of the nursing paradigm, in the way my job required me to practice nursing. The on-the-job medical education was interesting, and very complementary to my nursing training. But the dominant model of care I found myself hired to work under was medical care. As I grew in knowledge and proficiency, I found balance between the two and enjoyed the integration of both in my work. Over time, however, this medical paradigm encouraged, even merited, a 'name and tame' or a 'treat and street' way of streamlining and processing care. This was the attitude particularly when I worked in a teaching hospital. The medical students were being toughened for 'the practice of medicine.' There was almost an ego development training necessary to carry the responsibility they were to bear.

This conditioning is showing up in nurses as they become more medically knowledgeable, take on more responsibility, and are competing against the clock, the acuity and each other for praise from managers. This way may be necessary to meet the demands of a burdened system, but how much resulting undue stress, bullying and hints of dehumanization of the managers, staff or patients is acceptable?

Carolyn is a well-seasoned nurse. Being in her early sixties, she had difficulties finding suitable employment after being downsized from a cosmetic surgeon's office. After a challenging search through many online job opportunities, she was hired to work in an outpatient day surgery center – another of her specialties. The nursing care came easily to her. She found it interesting how they managed the work flows and learned to appreciate the differences in policies and procedures between facilities. The pace of the workflow required her to hone her efficiency skills, because one slight delay could lead to a backlog that lasted the rest of her work shift. As she was juggling the coming and going of patients and their treatments, she approached a patient's bed to help them reposition onto their side. The patient showed that she had the strength to do it on her own, so Carolyn saved herself a few steps by not walking completely to her bedside. The pole and infusion pump crashed down onto the bed. Carolyn felt horrible and responsible. Luckily the patient was just startled and uninjured. Carolyn could only think of how she had felt rushed. Normally she would have confirmed the infusion lines were free from entanglement while directly assisting with the turn.

Carolyn spoke with her manager and said she truly questioned that this job was for her. She told her manager that this environment was exactly what she avoided her entire career. Being forced to rush to the extent that she could jeopardize patient safety and having to give more of her attention to the computer than her patients contributed to the compromise in foundational nursing care. The manager confirmed. "Yes, my younger nurses have the energy and can handle the pace and technology. But they call in sick a lot, are less thorough and seem less motivated to be at the bedside. My older nurses don't like the pace and have a harder time with the computers. But their experience, knowledge, dependability and integrity are very valuable." Her manager pleaded, "Please stay, I need you."

Consider and answer these questions in your journal:
> What paradigm stress do you find in the above story for Carolyn, her manager, the patients or yourself?
> What are the similarities and disparities you experience between the paradigm under which you were educated as a nurse and the one you were hired to work in?
> What is stressful about the disparities between the two paradigms for you?
> Which elements of what you described are yin and which are yang?
> How do the practices and philosophies of nurses you work with differ? Compare the nurses who have careers that are both longer and shorter than yours.
> How were you prepared by your nursing program to work in the business of healthcare and for task-oriented productivity?
> When did you last decide how to provide care via the nursing process?
> When were you last merited for implementing a successful nursing plan of care for a patient?
> How is the therapeutic environment between nurse and patient established, maintained and supported in your job?
> As she left work on her last day, a colleague who retired more than a decade ago said, "I don't do conveyor belt nursing." What would she think today?

If your experience has revealed a variety or realizations and situations, write a description of how your paradigm has changed during your career.

» What changes do you feel good about and how would you improve others?

» Do you measure any correlation between the subsequent changes in your personal and work paradigms during your career and your level of stress?

A phenomenon occurs when people are limited in the practice of their beliefs and truths. Eventually, they'll give up their own thoughts. They will join the dominant thought system, likely in the name of survival – forgetting how they used to see things. This is a sensitive but realistic subject.

The medical model has elevated nurses in knowledge and standing. However, this came at a price. It also gave nurses a steady increase in responsibility, hence more risk. With less emphasis on nursing theory of care and greater reward for applying the new information, nurses could forget their own values and philosophies as the other replaces them. Nurses need their paycheck so they do what their jobs demands, but much of what they are complaining about today as stressful seems to stem from a parting from values. I do not intend this as a dualistic challenge to assign blame. It is to magnify the potential milieu, keeping in mind the important role of environment and the Yin-Yang relationship of things.

In the last decade, I have known several nurses who have pursued becoming a Nurse Practitioner (NP). Most have answered the same when I asked how they like their education and new role… "It is okay, but it is not what I thought it would be." I find it interesting this is the same comment new nurses often make at the beginning of their career. The NPs further said, "They want us to think like a doctor. I thought I would be doing nursing."

This can be another stress for nurses. It is likely more subtle, a deep generalized dissatisfaction or fatigue because the suppression of feelings and emotions uses immense energy. In the current medical model, the mind is treated as if separate from the body and symptoms, as if uninfluenced by thoughts, feelings and emotions. We should recall Candace Pert's statement in Chapter 4 about psychosomatic illness and wellness, and that emotions have power to influence health. There is an important capacity that people who are nurses inherently bring into their roles. Consider that the *Soul* is integral to nursing care. The medical model of learned knowledge is at best elusive on this subject. You are the *Soul,* patients are the *Soul,* as are the other people working for the patient's good. The job, its duties, the technology, and treatments are personas, tools, and mechanisms. Technology can improve the efficiency to some extent. But qualified professional people with *Soul* are necessary to administer and support treatments, procedures, and medications humanely. It's true that efficiency is important for the bottom line of the business behind it all. The question is whether this equation contains any sustainable remnant of the important variable of *Soul.*

> (♥) Recall a *Soul-to-Soul* moment you have had with a patient.
> How did you know that you were *Soul-to-Soul?* What did
> you give? What did you receive? How did it make you feel?
> How often do you have this experience with a patient?
> How long does it take to get *Soul-to-Soul* with a patient?
> Were there any lingering effects for you? How important
> is this connection for your patients? How important is
> this connection for you? How does this type of connection
> affect your stress levels and level of job satisfaction? Write
> your answers and explore other thoughts in your journal.

The amazing thing about *Soul* time is that in the time to connect and share, it can *shift* an attitude, the outcome of a treatment, the trajectory of the day, or productivity – so the payoff can be well worth it.

As you made notes in your journal in the above Heart Activity, did you feel any change in the area of your heart while you considered your experiences of intimacy, warmth, a hand squeeze, a smile, a lean, a laugh, a hug, a thank you? This is the payout that keeps on giving, especially for you, the number-one trusted professional.[18] You are meaningful and purposeful because of your irreplaceable value as the conduit of care. When you understand your stress, its sources and your experiences, you can become empowered and more influential.

Being a part of the yin and the yang of the medical care culture, nurses are in a unique position to lead the cultural transformation need-ed to address the complexity of stressors and their impact on well-being and health. We cannot create health with the same level of thinking, lifestyle, or toxicity that created illness. Nurses know a lot about caring for and promoting health. However, that knowledge may be fuzzy or seem less relevant because it differs from the respected, skilled training to give treatments for illness. The two dovetail, but there needs to be more balance – a partnership in which nurses lead with their knowledge and wisdom. Your stress is motivating you to get back in touch with yourself and your nursing knowledge, so you will influence this cultural shift with wisdom from your stress.

In the article, "Leading the Shift from a Dominator to a Partner-ship Culture," the authors encourage this concept individually and col-lectively. They suggest that each time we do one of the following we contribute to the creation of such a culture:

- Discernment instead of judgment
- Appreciation over criticism
- Generosity in place of self-interest
- Reconciliation over retaliation[19]

Imagine for a minute this culture they describe. How would this change your workplace? Does imagining this culture ease the breath you were holding, relax your fore-head, release your shoulders, or maybe calm the feeling in your gut? Make notes in your journal.

What do you like about this concept? Dislike? What ideas does it bring up for you? Fears? Options? Is there any calling for you? Are you starting to sense that you are the heart of health care? Can you see that by working with your experience of stress, you might regain the energy and clarity to *shift* things toward health within yourself, your family, your work and health culture? Add your thoughts about these questions to your journal.

After reading and soul searching about stress in the prior pages, it needs emphasizing that your subjective interpretation of any environment, situation, interaction or comment is most important when it comes to the impact it might have for you. At a minimum, you could attribute this to the powerful placebo and nocebo effects.[20] However, it can also be because you are the creator of your reality (experience) through your interpretations, both judgmental and optimistic. This is a foundational concept of The Perceived Stress Scale developed by Sheldon Cohen and his colleagues in 1983, which remains in use today.[21]

Do the self assessment of perceived stress. Find this classic stress assessment tool in the online book support materials at . It asks about your thoughts and feelings, and their frequency during the prior month. The result takes into consideration the importance of your perception of what is happening in your life. What surprises you about the results? Make notes in your journal.

New Science Confirms Old Wisdom of Stress and Healing

As the craftsman handed over the handmade wooden massage table, his parting words were memorable, "A healing of one being is a healing of all beings." It was beautiful... the table and the quote. He imbued the table with his creative energy and love. As a new massage therapist in 1987, I felt I would soothe away much stress, strain and pain working on this table. This was an altar for bodywork. I coveted that quote; it touched me and it sounded nice. I wasn't sure I fully understood it, but it felt true and I wanted to understand it.

It did not take long for me to realize that before I could help another relax or heal I had to relax and be in a healing space and not hurried, stressed, hungry or otherwise diverted from that person. As a massage therapist, my work was to hold the space for the highest good to occur for the one beneath my hands. I came to understand and live by this philosophy. I adopted a similar intent in my nursing career.

Over time, gaining more work experience and confidence facilitates an inner calm. However, as your experience of stress may indicate, the demands of the increasing complexity and tempo of the medical paradigm of your job can challenge your inner calm. Learning to be at ease, alert, and resilient is of utmost importance to retain a human connection between self and patient, and balance the external counter-strain.

It is said the longest distance is from the head to the heart. Medicine and nursing require critical thinking and accurate, efficient decision-making skills. It is easy to function predominantly from this potent intellectual prowess which is distancing from a patient. Cultivating *heart* will both sharpen cognitive skills and balance them with yin qualities. The result is a warmer, healing relationship and improved outcome for the patient. Can you see the yin and yang forces at work? Do you see how the role of a nurse, in relationship to mainstream medicine, is to bring and cultivate both heart and health? You are the heart that rocks health care. Your purpose is to flourish, influence and lead from your heart, in relationship to a healthcare system that fixes what mishaps occur. You and your colleagues are in a model as defined by your job description, but your biggest role is up to you to fulfill.

The bio-technology and achievements of modern medicine are revered worldwide. When a mangled body presents in the ED, the trauma surgeon's skill is phenomenal at repairing and putting things back together. In cardiac and cerebrovascular events, medical and technological interventions are astounding. Resuscitative science and medicine are reviving people and restoring them to a fully functional condition by stopping the insult and supporting reversal of damage. All those involved in medicine, including nurses, can appreciate the honor of being a part of these amazing specialized successes.

In contrast, medical management of chronic and debilitating disease is episodic and symptomatic, and often less successful than with acute injuries and illnesses. This method of treatment attempts to systemize its delivery sometimes without the mindful attention needed to determine the root cause, intervene, and allow the body systems to reverse such a condition. Further, the system of medical care is overburdened, and it is becoming apparent that it cannot handle the volume of people with these chronic and debilitating diseases. Despite innovative drugs, their side effects may contribute to the need for further or more complex medical care.[22] As described, healthcare is predominately a yang system. It screens to detect symptoms of illness for early treatment, but is lagging in health assessment and health promotion. This is not the same as screening for early illness detection, rather it assesses and supports the vitality and efficiency of pathways, and identifies environmental factors that may challenge these such as toxins, stress and lack of nutrients. Chemistry and classic physics are the basis of the mainstream medical model. This science is used in a reductionistic, mechanistic and compartmentalized manner. It looks at the body metaphorically as a machine. It has its applications but foundationally accepts that there is minimal to no connection or influence between systems, let alone between people. But have you heard that "the whole is greater than the sum of its parts"?

There is another dimension from which to view and approach stress, health and healing – the quantum perspective. In 1918, Max Planck earned Nobel Prize recognition for advancing physics with his discovery of quanta. Niels Bohr, a Danish physicist and Nobel Prize winner in Physics in 1922, said, "If quantum mechanics hasn't profoundly shocked you, you haven't understood it yet."[23] This relationship-based science has become the basis of modern physics though it is not yet adopted into the mainstream practice of medicine. The quantum model explains the nature and behavior of matter and energy as *shifting* states of quanta, which are packets of light.[24]

This is significant because this theory also reveals energy fields, unity and human potential. This is likely different from what you were taught in physics and physiology. But perhaps it is like some nursing theories from nursing school, such as Martha Roger's "The Science of Unitary Human Beings."[25]

Despite the existence of ancient medicinal and healing systems that have been cultivating health in certain cultures for thousands of years, these nursing theories are not likely put into practice or have much value placed upon them in your job. Despite current research proving the soundness of those cultural approaches, mainstream medicine has been slow to adopt influence from quantum physics even as it continues to influence technological advancement. In the 21st Century, preventative, holistic, and integrated healthcare is the direction we must move into. It has been said, "The healing of a patient must include more than the biology and chemistry of their physical body; by necessity, it must include the mental, emotional, and spiritual (energetic) aspects."[26]

Adapting quantum principles and energy "depends on the ability of allopathic medicine to merge physics with biochemistry."[27] You may ask, "Why the slow integration of this perspective?" We would do well to balance that question with another, "What if they integrated it? Asking "Why" and "What if" questions are mind-widening and help bring about change in the world around you according to Warren Berger, author of *A More Beautiful Question.*[28] The answers would challenge the system to change. This system views everything as alternative to its practices instead of all therapeutic systems, including allopathy, to be complementary. Holistically, nurses can lead the way with inquiry and wisdom through self-care application, the teaching of the cultivation of health and well-being, and facilitating healing in their families and communities. This will empower people to build health and make healthy choices with great potential of reducing chronic, lifestyle-related illnesses.

The Perfection of Imperfection

I hope that your thoughts, feelings, perhaps even principles and opinions are jarring from the review and activities in these first few chapters. Also that your creativity is stirring and that you sense light being shed on your experience of stress in your job and health. This movement of ideas and the wavering of rigid boundaries reduces the resistance that opposes change. You may experience a state of wonder or curiosity. The beginner's mind is a Zen concept of seeing something familiar and ordinary, as if for the first time. This is foundational to healing and innovation because of the many possibilities within the beginner's mind compare to the limited mind of an expert, as explained by Shunryu Suzuki in his book, *Zen Mind, Beginner's Mind.*[29]

Within the well-intended mainstream medical healthcare system and even within your plans of care for your patients' treatments, they are not perfect. There is a metaphorical crack, or flaw in everything, which is the perfection. It is the space for potential to exist as it lets in the light of possibility for creativity, healing and whatever is possible to occur. This concept resembles the meaning of the seed of the opposite contained within the Yin-Yang symbol... that of potential. So if you have a desire or even so much as a sense of the light of possibility, you have found the perfect crack from where you can open to what is possible and transform your stress, your health, and perhaps the care of health. Your desire, questioning, and seeking reveal a metaphorical hand-hold to leverage the creation of a new perspective, experience and reality. You can interpret this as another validation of that feeling you acknowledged at the start of this book... of that inner call light which needs your attention as it is showing you there is a crack, a space for potential.

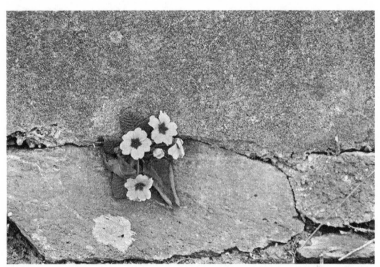

Public Domain Photo - adapted by Vivo Digital Arts

The awareness you gained and the cracks you have found through engaging in Part One of this book have hopefully provided some acknowledgement and are facilitating some relief. These incremental adjustments convert to significant changes in the bearings of your inner compass, which will be a guide toward the success you seek. Breathe with ease and prepare for the journey in Part Two with the following Heart Activity.

Say, "Ah, Success." Did you think it or whisper it to yourself? Now say it again, out loud while feeling the words. Do you feel any sensation, relief or empowerment? Notice any vibrations in your throat and chest, inhibitions or restrictions, your breath, facial expressions, shoulders, postures or sensations in your body as you spoke the words. You may not resonate with these words right away or you may feel disassociated or even resistant toward them. Be honest with yourself. Be who and as you are. Be in the experience.

Your feelings or absence of them are clues to guide you, so glean bits of information and meaning. Repeat "Ah, Success" aloud. What were your thoughts this time? Were your eyes open or closed? What was different when reading it to yourself versus saying it out loud? Make notes in your journal.

Use the A-B-Cs to shift your neurology and physiology to a more centered and stable state in the face of a non life-threatening situation or stress. As your emotions synchronize with your desired outcome, it will be even more effective. Managing the effects of stress with self-care techniques and strategies can be effective. But if the circumstances, environment or root causes stay the same, stress can still become unmanageable. Acknowledgment is important to stop the insanity of expecting the outcome to be different. You need to have a fresh perspective and a positive action plan to get more desirable results.

The AH SUCCESS Process can help you find other ways, means, options, solutions and dreams. It helps you move toward and draw closer to your success as you reduce the resistance and transform the blocks that seem to be in between. Choose one situation or stressor that is impacting your life to explore using the AH SUCCESS Process in Part Two.

PART TWO

AH SUCCESS

S tress, illness and conflict are fluid states or conditions, not static entities. They contain messages and information. This means you are not stuck in your experience of them. Leading edge science has proven that our universe is very interactive, as is your state of health. You must intentionally take part to accomplish what you want and bring about change. This is the quantum way to change your stress and involves changing your internal milieu via your response and relationship to it. This is best done by self-care and self-regulation of your physiology, such as using the *Easy as A-B-C Technique.*

Mahatma Gandhi, inspired and challenged, "You must be the change that you wish to see in the world." Whether you want to change the world, your job, your relationships or your stress, the courageous way to lead change is from within.

When you make a change, *a shift*, you influence those external things like people, situations and environments to shift. This is because of the inter-relatedness of all things.

In Part Two you learn how to accomplish this *shift* and more about the connected-ness of things, as you experience the AH SUCCESS Process. This evolutionary method will help you learn, adapt and evolve toward the well-being and personal empowerment you seek. It guides you on how to create within yourself the success you want to have in your relationships, your life and the world around you as an intentional part of its manifestation.

Below is a list of the nine steps in the AH SUCCESS Process.

The *AH SUCCESS* Process

A AWARENESS

H HOLD SPACE FOR POSITIVE POSSIBILITY

S SHIFT

U UNLOCK INNER WISDOM

C CENTER

C CHOOSE

E ELEVATE

S SEE YOURSELF WITH DESIRED RESULTS

S STEP INTO POSITIVE ACTION

The steps are progressive yet inter-connected. For instance, the concept of *awareness* is the first step, but permeates all the steps as they interrelate in intricate ways. This and other quantum forces have always been at work creating your health, relationships and life while you may not have been aware of their presence. You will learn that it is possible and beneficial to be active in directing those same forces on which the steps in the AH SUCCESS Process are based.

The Process is repeatable and you can use the skills and techniques with any issue, challenge, circumstance or relationship where understanding, insight, change and success are needed or desired. As you use the Process, the steps in will become simpler. You will also integrate knowledge and your wisdom from using them, making the Process your own as it becomes second nature. You will recognize moments that present you with an opportunity to choose how to think, act or self-regulate in order to influence your health and success, rather than feed stress. In these moments you will intuitively apply the step you need at the time you need it.

If you haven't already, choose the stressor that has your shoulders aching or keeps you awake at night. The exercises at the end of each chapter in this section will help you integrate the step-related concepts by applying them to your specific situation and advance you through the AH SUCCESS Process.

CHAPTER 6

AWARENESS

As awareness is key to success - it is the foundation of the AH SUC-CESS Process. This conceptual and transformational process evolved from and contains the mini meditation and self-regulation sequence called the Easy as A-B-C Technique that was introduced in Chapter 4. Both are rooted in and woven with *A-Awareness* as the foundation for success. The two concepts of *B-Breath* and *C-Center* in the A-B-Cs, are also shared with the Process. The A-B-C Technique, however, remains an independent, in-the-moment tool to reset your physiology whenever you feel stressed.

Michael Kitson, art historian, said of awareness, "If you have it, teach it. If you lack it, seek it." Your awareness will broaden and deepen with valuable conceptual and experiential understanding as you work through the AH SUCCESS Process.

The destination of this book can be whatever *you* seek as success. However the pursuit of success or any object of success can be challeng-ing and stressful because it engages attachment, which is counter to the purpose of this book. Success finds you as a result of your awareness and choices. First, in learning to *shift* out of an unnecessary stress response using the A-B-Cs. Second, in *real-izing* it through heart-synchronized thoughts, feelings, emotions, choices, and actions, using the resiliency-building skills in the AH SUCCESS Process.

This is an inward journey that creates internal milieu changes to influence success externally. It may seem paradoxical, but restoring your well-being becomes empowerment, which when cultivated, expresses into health, innovation, influence and leadership. In this perspective, answering your inner call light makes an ideal subject for your adventure through the Process.

(🖐) Since the A-B-C Technique facilitates awareness, it is helpful to do the technique in preparation for the Heart Activities and also as you consider new information. So feel free the use it as you're inclined, without prompts or instruction. This will help you be present with the new information, reinforce the process and gain experience-based knowledge of the concepts as we explore them more deeply.

Practice it now. Refer to Chapter 4 for a review or simply follow the prompts below and let your awareness, breath and center be your guide.

A is for Awareness:
Become aware and expand your awareness.
B is for Breath:
Follow your breath, slow and deepen it.
C is for Center:
Shift to your center.

Dwell within your center and become familiar with this space and yourself within it. You will likely let go of your breath – it will become effortless, shallow and slow while you are *centered*. When the experience feels complete, you are done.

How was this different from your prior experience with the A-B-Cs? What was familiar for you about this experience? Was it easier to become centered? What new characteristics of your center did you discover? Make any journal notes that you feel inclined to.

Awareness and Honesty

You have many expectations that come from the outside but the most important ones come from the person you see in the mirror. Someone's belief in or expectation of you can encourage something deep within you, but you must tend to the flame of desire and the belief in your own creativity for you to truly succeed. This is intimate, deep and requires honesty. It's okay to be where you are at any given moment and want to go where you want to go. However, success comes through the natural order of things which is about growth, not attainment. You must be as honest with yourself as you can and be willing to become more honest with yourself over time. Sometimes we know when we are stuck and sometimes we cannot get out of our own way. The honesty part involves our readiness, willingness and ability.

I give to you this affirmation I picked up along the way and have frequently told myself: "I'm always in the right place at the right time, engaged in the right activity." Within that is awareness and acceptance. For me, it is often accompanied by the desire to change that place, time or activity, or become what I want to become. Honesty with yourself will facilitate this. Another affirmation I tell myself when I think I know what I want: "This or something better." Why limit myself by my own notions?

	READY	*WILLING*	*ABLE*
TIME	*FR TH* *LW RH*	*FR TH* *LW RH*	*FR TH* *LW RH*
ANTICIPATORY	*FR TH* *LW RH*	*FR TH* *LW RH*	*FR TH* *LW RH*
SITUATIONAL	*FR TH* *LW RH*	*FR TH* *LW RH*	*FR TH* *LW RH*
ENCOUNTER	*FR TH* *LW RH*	*FR TH* *LW RH*	*FR TH* *LW RH*

Ready Willing Able chart

Let's take your *temperature* to raise your awareness about how fired up you are with readiness for regaining your vitality. This is real power that can be transformational and differs from impulsive motivation. Above is a suggested chart format to draw on a journal page for recording your answers. Rate how you feel in this moment for the three areas of being – Ready, Willing and Able. Do this for your experience of each of the four main types of work stress discussed in the previous chapter. These four types of stress are: Time, Anticipatory, Situational and Encounter. Use this scale: Frozen, Thawing, Luke Warm and Red Hot. Circle your answers and write the other information from this activity in your journal.

How do you know that you are ready? What tells you your answer? Do you get any feeling or sensation? What part does willingness have in readiness? What determines ability for you? What limits it?

What would it be like if you were a degree warmer in any of these areas? What would it feel like? What would it take to move you up a degree in each of the areas that need some warming to increase your readiness? It is okay to be where you are, but notice if you get stuck at a particular temperature. Awareness of this may help to increase your fire of desire to transform your attitude, experience, situation, circumstance and stress levels. Write your answers and illuminations.

Willingness on your part is most necessary. Sometimes willingness can exceed your preparedness. Other times, you must challenge yourself to jump the hurdles of perceived limitations in your mind. Still other times it oozes through a gap in logic or space between rules. The gap or space is the 'crack' introduced in Chapter 5, the imperfection that lets in the light of possibility – this time showing up as willingness. When willingness meets a new perspective more things become possible. You can influence and even change your current circumstance or experience from what presents in this space, especially in the presence of willingness.

In the willing act of considering a possibility, visualizing what it would feel and be like, you have begun the process of creating or *realizing* it. This is because *your* thought, feelings and emotion creates the physiology of *your* experience, which is *your* reality. Your new experience, will bring awareness to motivate your willingness.

> In the same context of your stress, are you willing? What does it feel like to be willing? Explore what you need in order to cultivate willingness. Revisit the previous Heart Activity and spend time feeling warmer in those areas that are calling for it, perhaps by adding willingness. Make notes to prompt yourself of how to increase your readiness with willingness.

Ability is a mental, emotional, physical and spiritual capacity. Often external circumstances define ability, sometimes the determination is made internally determination. What is your measure of ability: muscle strength, money, beauty, knowledge, or by virtue of integrity, fortitude or conscientiousness?

> Continuing with the same context of your stress, are you able? Do you *know* you are able, *decide* you are able, or do you make a choice to be? List what makes you able. Write another list of what else you *need* to be able. Now look over this second list and circle the ones that you are able to do something about to prepare, condition, train for, or otherwise acquire in order to improve your *ability*. Now prioritize them. Were you aware of these things and conditions you perceive as necessary? Awareness enhances your ability to create, change, and attain. What new understanding have you gained about the relationships between readiness, willingness and ability? Add notes about your new insights to your journal.

Dimensions of Awareness

Awareness is multidimensional. It is a state that involves mind, body and environmental use of attention, perception and the senses. It can be experienced as a state and exist as a realm. As a state it has qualities such as expansive, focused or absent. As a realm, it can be any of the following: self-awareness, cultural awareness, heart awareness, health awareness, global awareness or spiritual awareness.

Do you ever unplug, vacate or space out during boredom, pain, conflict, stress or overwhelm? This response can be concerning, protective, relaxing or creative. Think of times when someone was talking to you and you were completely unaware, or during a conversation when you drifted off and had to ask the other person to repeat a detail. It can be embarrassing in a casual conversation, rude when a patient is telling their story, detrimental in a job interview and even dangerous when you drive home from work without remembering the journey. These situations can show you need relief, space or to increase your presence through awareness.

Where do *you* go in these situations? What part of *you* leaves? Your awareness is what leaves and what allows you to notice this happening. How do you experience awareness? Where is awareness for you? You will need to discover this answer for yourself. It is important to develop your ability to use awareness and to follow your inner guidance.

Become relaxed and allow your breath to be easy. Find your awareness. Is it in your right great toe? In your skin? Your gut? Your brain? See if it helps to have your eyes open or closed while locating it. How are you breathing while you are discovering?

Can your awareness be in a place other than where you are? Or other than where your body is? If you feel that you need to get up and walk around looking for it, go ahead.

At work, where is your awareness? Is it in the room with your patient? Is it in the pharmacy checking on the medications you are waiting for? Is it with you on your drive home?

Where did you find your awareness to be? *Did* you find your awareness? Make notes about your discoveries in your journal and describe your awareness. Revisit this activity and your discoveries when you want to explore further.

For success, you must learn to tend to the realms of self and inner awareness that involve being an honest friend to yourself. This is a way of *being* that connects and brings more awareness into the sub-conscious mind and body, and into your choices, actions, aspirations. It is a way of becoming familiar with your nature and the nature of your mind and personality – a way of becoming more authentic.

Awareness and Heart

The heart seems to be a place in the body where we show up – as in show up *for real*. Matters of the heart are not a job for autopilot. They are something that only we can show up for, appreciate, feel and do with full awareness. Your presence comes from within your heart where only you dwell. If you do not show up, it is eventually apparent because 'your heart isn't in it.' There is a sense of absenteeism. In this way, technology and artificial intelligence are pale approximations of human intelligence, creativity, intuition, compassion and innate abilities.

Where are you right now? Did you immediately think, here? Try it this way. Draw your fingers into a fist with your index finger pointing outward, use it to point to yourself as you say "me." Where are you pointing? What would you call that place? The most common result I have seen is people point to the center of their chest and associate that 'me-point' with their heart. Try saying "me" while pointing to other parts of your body, the chair or any place in the room. Does it feel awkward or did you find yourself elsewhere? Part of feeling loved by another is they 'see you.'

What is it they see? Love yourself first by using awareness to know yourself, your own heart. Write in your journal about your discoveries and experiences about locating *you*.

What relationship is there between your center and where you are? For many nurses, the heart is the center they find with the Easy as A-B-C Technique. Often when in your center – 'centered' – you feel more like yourself. Is it surprising that *you* may be found in your center, the still space within to dwell for stress relief, clarity, balance, connection, power and insight? Since the mind is where confusion, insecurity and fear happen, there is encouragement to use this technique with your mind-focused yet heart-centered work.

You will discover more about your center each time you go there. As we progress through the steps of the AH SUCCESS Process, keep this in mind: The heart of the matter is a matter of heart, because the heart matters.

By taking things to heart in the heart activities, you are tapping into your personal wisdom and courageously inventorying your thoughts, reactions and results, while increasing your awareness through your heart. This is possible because the heart has its own intelligence.

When neurons fire, electrical signals are transmitted along at high speed. As you process the information, have an idea or insight, your brain lights up with electricity, blood flow and oxygen. The light of awareness brings new perspectives and dispels myths that you unknowingly believed which blocked your success. Truths are revealed which can help you regain your vitality. You may feel like you already somehow know some of the information or are merely recalling forgotten knowledge as these truths dawn on your conscious mind. This is because you are *re-member-ing*, a process of *re-joining* or *re-connecting* with information you already know on a deep level – and the 'light bulb' turns on.

When you feel separate, isolated or alone – whether from yourself, a situation, information or another person – you can find connection *in light of it* or by taking it to heart. Light symbolizes awareness, possibility, consciousness and life. By using the A-B-Cs to seek a common ground with a person, situation or a part of your personality, you are seeking light in which to connect. Regardless of the mental, emotional or social *appearance* of differences, this illumination is in all.

In the privileged encounters that I've had, with the gift of a heart transplant recipient sharing stories of their post-transplantation neuro-sensory and emotional experiences, they shared the cravings, perceptions, urges, feelings, and emotions experienced since their transplants. It is most interesting that their doctors prescribed medications for anxiety and often made psychiatric referrals, when many times the person just wanted someone to listen and explore with them. Most were certain these were not their own and were from the organ donor; heart research supports this.

Interestingly, the heart is an organ of awareness, communication, emotion, and energy generation that is potent, intelligent and rejuvenating. It spontaneously generates electrical impulses and creates an electrical field measured 60 times greater than that of the brain by electrocardiogram (ECG) and electroencephalogram (EEG).[1] It is also the strongest magnetic field generator in the body is the heart, 5000 times greater than that of the brain and detectable up to six feet and more from the body.[2] This information makes it no wonder when you become present and aware – centered – you magnify your intuition, understanding and connection.

Further, the heart has endocrine functions, has its own nervous system, it thinks, feels and has its own memory. This heart intelligence is what contributes to the reported experiences of the heart transplant recipients, though there is valuable inter-system communication lost on other levels due to the severance of the vagus nerve. Significant to the experience of stress, the adaptive beat-to-beat variability is unable to occur without the vagal nerve feedback, resulting in a higher resting heart rate due to loss of vagal tone. The heart is left vulnerably sensitive to adrenaline, epinephrine, caffeine and other stimulants, making self-regulation even more valuable. Whereas, the native heart is connected to all the organs in the body via the autonomic nervous system and sends more information signals to the brain about the body's well-being, than the brain does to the body. This communication happens in four major ways:

1.   Neurologically via the transmission of nerve impulses
2.   Biochemically via hormones and neurotransmitters
3.   Biophysically which entails pressure waves
4.   Energetically via its electromagnetic field and interactions.

These are four potential pathways to intentionally influence the influence of stress and emotional signals when you feel stressed.[3] You truly were born with innate ability to influence your body, its inner pharmacy, and its electrical, emotional, neurochemical, immune and hormonal systems. Awareness of theses channels and learning to work with them are empowering components of self-care.

Neurocardiology studies the constant communication between the heart and the brain, and bioelectric studies relate to the electric language of the body primarily via the vagus nerve. These sciences are validating the body's ability to heal itself, and changing the course of diseases from cardiovascular to cancer.[4,5] Science and medicine are advancing into the use of *bio-regulation* for healing which merits your self-directed use of *self bio-regulation* for maintaining, building and restoring balance and health within your body.

Please have patience and understanding for yourself as you learn. Becoming more aware and engaging in heart-centered living are new habits to form while decreasing the automatic tendency to *logical-ize* everything. When practicing awareness and self-regulation techniques, it may require more time than your instant gratification brain expects. It is like training at the gym. Despite delayed results, the feeling of engagement is gratifying. As you become tone and fit of mind, emotions and awareness, you will gain more flexibility, agility and resilience. You may find that new options present and some old ways will no longer serve you. When living from your heart, you will more easily reset emotionally and activate energetic pathways to enhance performance in challenging or distracting situations, both at home and while on the job.

ⓜ What it look like if you used the Easy as A-B-Cs? How would things be different if you did deep breathing and centering before the start of your shift, following an emergency or an amygdala hijack? How would increasing awareness about your sense of well-being influence your self care, energy level, mental clarity, communication with your colleagues? Imagine the effects. How would you personally benefit from more awareness and heart energy? Is your heart still in your work? Record your thoughts on these questions.

As you work with your awareness and through the A-B-Cs and AH SUCCESS Process, the more heart-centered you will become. Then you will naturally seek to create heart-based connections and opportunities in health, work and life, which inherently builds influence. Can you open to this possibility?

Awareness and Becoming the Observer

Scientifically, observation is the mental act of placing your attention and gathering specific data. Observing your breath with awareness is noticing *what is,* without judgement. The ability to observe something means you are not that thing. That may sound simplistic, but stay with me to see why it is important to distinguish. That being said, it is powerful to realize the observer can influence what is observed, even in a scientific experiment.

I will share with you an exercise I experienced in the 1980s that is still effective. I do not know nor could I locate the source or author to whom I am extremely grateful. This was mind opening for me and I hope you find it helpful.

Get into a comfortable position and close your eyes, breathe and relax. Imagine a big, clear plastic bag. See it filling with beautiful colored light of your choice. Watch the swirls of light billow as the bag lofts and expands. You can make the bag as big as you would like. Now put your job into the bag, along with your title and responsibilities. Put your car into the bag. Add your house, your wardrobe and cosmetics. Put your problems in the bag, your worries, bills, health challenges, arguments, conflicts, losses and stressors. Watch as each thing takes up space inside the bag. Put your birthday in the bag, your educational degrees, titles, merits and trophies. Put any possession or problem you have into the bag – your clutter, the leaves that need raking, the laundry, even your boss or that traffic ticket. Put anything else you want into the bag...anything good or bad, happy or sad. Stuff it full and make it bigger if needed. Stuff it with your stuff.

When you feel you are done, look at the bag. Look at the things in the bag and see their colors and shapes, and the meanings they have for you. Take your time with this. Step back from the bag and look at all the things in the bag. The things are all there in the bag. You are not in the bag. You are not the bag. You are not the things in the bag. You are looking at the things in the bag. Who are you? Breathe and know who you are. When you have finished your experience, breathe deeply and bring your awareness to an open page in your journal. Write about your experience, what you learned about your identity and discovered about who you are.

Because it is too easy to blur the identify *of* yourself into identifying *with* a problem, stressor or emotion, this is important to discern. The ability to separate your responses from the influence of the drama or stress can help improve your *response-ability*. What you discovered may reveal a safe space between you, your burdens and the material world.

Awareness and Meditation

Meditation is a way of exploring awareness more deeply. After considering your own awareness, you may be curious what meditation has revealed to some of my clients about awareness. Though many initially guess their awareness is in their brain, they do not find it there. With practice, they each had similar discoveries, some of which are listed below:

1. Awareness is found most easily, at first, in stillness.
2. Awareness seems to be in between, within or surrounding, as opposed to at a specific location.
3. Awareness seems to be present even when I think I am pre-occupied.

Awareness is something primordial. The is in contrast to the mental focus necessary for your job, it is much more fundamental. You can learn facts and procedures, like how to plant and water a garden, and there you go it's done. However, successful blooms and fruit require tending to the balance of life-giving elements and nutrients, pruning and weeding which are about cultivation. You rarely get permission, let alone are taught how to tend to yourself, your health, in this way. Meditation is one such way. It will bring your awareness way beyond the list: eat right, exercise, stay hydrated, get sleep, reduce stress, etc.

Getting beyond the directives and demands of daily life and work is a skill necessary for vibrant health. You do not have your own nurse tending to your every need. In our culture, one does not get one until they are sick and even then someone else has to authorize it. So guess what? It is up to you to take care of yourself including body, *being* and health, After becoming aware of your well-being, you can influence a *shift* amongst your family and colleagues that provides a culture of support for self-care, health and success.

Becoming more aware is an intentional, participatory process. Meditation is a skill and practice that can easily and progressively be developed for cultivating awareness and calming the mind.

Soften your gaze. Allow your mind to drift. Accept any noises and hums around you as invitations to go deeper and beyond. Notice how the noises are *there* and you are *here*. Bring your awareness to your breath, which is *here* with you, and observe. Awareness follows breath. If your awareness doesn't *shift* to your breathing by your intention, place a hand over the center of your chest. This is gentle training for your awareness because it also follows touch.

This is in part why touch is important in the healing relationship with your patients, even when they seem absent in a coma or when they are dying. Your touch affirms, connects and communicates with their awareness, bringing yours to meet it.

Feel the air movement in and out of your nose. Follow it through the sinuses, throat and windpipes. Feel your lungs inflate and deflate. Reposition your hand from your chest to your abdomen. Move the air in and out from here. How does your breath change? What changes do you notice in the movements and feelings of breathing? Is there a change in your satisfaction from each breath?

As you notice, follow, feel, observe, what is it that shifts around, leaving one experience to move on and observe the next? It is your awareness that is moving about. You use your attention, which is of the mind, throughout a workday to focus and respond. Attention follows the eyes. Notice the difference between attention and awareness. Is it possible to have your attention on one thing while being aware of something else? Make notes in your journal.

Amidst the *busy-ness* of your life and the *busi-ness* of your job, you must learn to go beyond your thoughts to stay in touch with yourself on a deep level. The cues and feedback from the outside world are plentiful and easily distracting of your attention. Your body automatically responds to those cues with bio-hormonal, neurochemical and electromagnetic processes of thought, feeling and emotion which, in turn, affect your health. Only you can tend to this inner terrain through awareness by caring for your inner environment and source of health.

Awareness and Mindfulness

Mindfulness is a way of using awareness to care for this inner terrain by stabilizing turbulence in your mind. The illusion of fullness of the mind is comprised of thoughts, both conscious and unconscious.

As you become aware of these things, you also become aware that you are observing them and can interact with them. As you observe, you will also find space between your thoughts, emptiness, or *no-thing-ness,* and it is in this gap where you can find rest and pure awareness. This emptiness is what the fullness is made of in mindfulness. When doing activities with mindfulness, the activity is met with your awareness. Your awareness can merge with the *doing,* become *being,* and this is when you can achieve *flow.* Athletes, artists, musicians, meditators and healers know and revel in this state, some calling it 'in the zone.'

In this mindfulness meditation, slow thoughts and calm your body. First, ask yourself what is haunting you? Perhaps thoughts about going to work the next day, bills stacking up and other obligations are cluttering your mind during your time off.

Close your eyes and become aware that you are having such thoughts. As the observer, hear them, watch them racing in your mind, and notice any body sensations associated with them. These are your reactions to the experience of these thoughts. You can change your thoughts by will, listen for meaning, or breathe and let these distressing thoughts pass as you *shift* into the space for inner ease.

If you'd like, follow these suggestions. Become aware of a cuddly pet or animal lying beside you. Feel the smile warming your face, dissolving the tension of concern in your forehead, brow and jaw as you look at your pet. Look deep into their eyes. Feel your desire to reach out and pet her. Feel the intention in your mind. Notice your shoulders release any work-related tension. There is a gentle lifting contraction of your deltoid, then extension of your arm as you move to connect your hand with your furry friend. Hover your palm moving slowly toward your pet. Close your eyes and notice when you first sense her presence under your hand. Is it a tingle or warmth? Pause at your first sensation of fur. Feel your hand melt into her fur and sense

> her being absorbing your touch. Rest in the furry, cozy connection. What changes in your being and body during this connection?
>
> As you observe in this way with your awareness completely in the present, your experience magnifies and the connection becomes the only thing in your awareness. Bring your hand into your lap and experience your own relaxed, buoyant being. What is left when you have found the stillness and quiet? Make notes in your journal.

Enjoying a connection with a pet is restful and restorative to a stressed nurse. The separation from work and related thoughts by engaging in mindfulness is balancing to the mind and energy. You are the master of your awareness.

The National Center for Complementary and Integrative Health (NCCIH) says, "Research supports that meditation can reduce blood pressure, symptoms of irritable bowel syndrome, anxiety, depression and insomnia...flare-ups in people who have had ulcerative colitis... [and] has a long history of use for increasing calmness and physical relaxation, improving psychological balance, coping with illness, and enhancing overall health and well-being."[6] Mindfulness meditation study findings support "that a short program in mindfulness meditation produces demonstrable effects on brain and immune function... [and] suggest that meditation may change brain and immune function in positive ways."[7] All things connect via your energetic neurobiology. Meditation and mindfulness raise awareness for self regulation. (i)

Awareness and Consciousness

The concepts of awareness and consciousness are often used in conversation casually, as if interchangeable. They remain a bit fuzzy even in scholarly or research oriented writing as scientists venture to gain more understanding. Because of this, I suggest getting an understanding of the way they are defined by that writer or researcher and then follow their flow to understand the point they are making. I hope to establish a flow of understanding for the AH SUCCESS Process. Despite my efforts to describe and define them for you, their fluid nature makes research and the definitions blurry. That is why the Heart Activities and application in your life are most important. My words may fall short, but your experience is what you have to learn from and guide you.

While attention is triggered by sensory processing in the brain, awareness is both *looming* as it arises from within and intentional as it can expand at will. Awareness involves sensing and brings a more spacious and expansive dimension of knowing thorough observation and intention.

The following inter-related conceptual perspectives about consciousness may help you approach understanding. There are medical and psychological perspectives of being *conscious* as a process of the brain being awake and in a level of alertness or wakefulness. It also can refer to a state of mind, where one can think and reason, and includes the ability to deal with abstracts like symbols, metaphors and jokes. *Consciousness,* as it is primarily explored here, is an innate and spontaneous or intelligence, the source of which is greater than your mind and body. It is absolute whereas the levels described as waking, thinking, dreaming and sleep are relative. Perception of this level can detect subtleties of presence, energy, and essence – beyond your own thoughts, feelings and emotions. This is the level of awareness we are honing.

This is something to do when you are waking from sleep. Naturally awakening without an alarm is ideal. Read through this to become familiar with it so you can recall it. Imagine experiencing it as you read.

Upon your initial stirring in the morning, prior to opening your eyes, dwell there in the depths of altered consciousness. Your mind is clear of thoughts, you may be aware that you had a dream and be able to recall it. *Where* are you in this experience? *What* are you – consciousness, awareness, mind? *Have* you begun to notice your body yet? Notice the words denoting possession: *your* stirring, *your* eyes, *your* mind, *you had* a dream, *your* body. You have these things, but are they you? Did you find yourself? Did you find *you*? What is the difference between *you* and yourself?

The insights from my clients about awareness that were listed in the prior section show that they experienced being aware of the presence of consciousness within and around themselves. For you, what showed up first, *you* or consciousness? When did *you* become *aware*? Was it before your mind became conscious? Consciousness is present despite awareness. It precedes awareness, before thought, before *you* connect with your body. Where are *you* in all of this? You cannot know if the body is conscious until you become aware of it. To be aware of it, you cannot be the body, but rather *be in* the body. There is a mirroring or reflective quality to awareness. If consciousness is already present and then lit by your awareness, you experience it in your body. It is like you are looking at yourself in a mirror and becoming self-aware. Which are you...the body or the reflection, or the one occupying the body and observing the reflection? This reflective state is *conscious awareness* or *being consciously aware*.

Feel the energy and awareness shift as you pause after saying each of these words: me, my, I, and I am. Your experience may be enhanced by adding an object such as, my hand. *You* are the pilot of the body. Is that the *me* or *I* version of *you*? When *you* engage the body's instruments (senses, organs, systems), *you* feel aware and experience as the body. Contemplate this. Make notes about your experience and observations; include questions for further study.

Awareness can be turned on and off as if by a switch, when you zone in or out. But consciousness is not limited to the body, it is omnipresent, including within the body, as long as the body is inspiring (*in-spirit-ing*) and until it expires (*ex-spirits*) for the last time. Respiration (*re-spirit-ation*) is the cyclical re-connection with spirit, consciousness.

Awareness of this is an important self regulation skill. If *you* are willing to honor consciousness within, you will increase your *response-ability*, health, empowerment, and influence. You will also be able to honor it in others.

Awareness and Breathing

Breathing is a natural guide for your awareness and *vehicle of consciousness*. It has expansive qualities and the ability to move things such as your awareness, oxygen and energy in the body. Sometimes we may control our breathing, but most of the time it is unconscious. The characteristics of the breath, such as depth, rate and pattern, respond to the influence of being cold, relaxed, stressed and of your thought. The momentum of thinking and breathing paces our experience. Erratic thoughts during anxiety are accompanied by a shallow rapid breathing pattern, irregular heart beats and chaotic physiology. When breathing with awareness, it neutralizes stress, brings clarity, focus and healthy physiology

When nervous, the diaphragm – the muscle doing the work of breathing – tenses and cannot regulate breathing properly. In today's productivity driven culture, it is common to chronically control air movement, volume, pitch and diction using the chest and throat muscles, which are less efficient. This also drives the sympathetic feedback, adding fuel to the fiery effects of stress. Compounded by a sedentary lifestyle, poor diet, toxins, medications, emotions and stress, there is severe negative influence on the tonicity of the vagus nerve. Resetting and promoting the responsiveness of your vagus nerve is important for building, recovering and maintaining health, and resiliency. If you are starting to see a relationship between stress, perception, brain function, breathing, the autonomic nervous system and vagus nerve, it will be easier for you to accept vagal nerve activity as a potent tool for healing.[8] Also, the honing of self-awareness and skills of self-regulation, such as breathing, grant access to these benefits of stimulating and healing your vagus nerve.

Abdominal or diaphragmatic breathing is proper breathing and parasympathetic inducing. It is beneficial while doing your job because of the dominant cognitive demands. As you breathe deeper, slower and more fully from your abdomen, you can benefit from the parasympathetic influence of the vagus nerve, including improved mental focus. Breathing this way has many other benefits such as massaging the abdominal organs, toning pelvic muscles, and improving core stability and strength. Research specifically reveals "the vagus nerve inhibits oxidative stress, inflammation and sympathetic activity (and associated hypoxia)...current non-invasive methods exist to activate this nerve for neuro-modulation, and have promising clinical effects."[9] Here in lies power for your self regulation, recuperation from stress, and physiological reset because of the vagus nerve's "...regulation of metabolic homeostasis, [a] key role in the neuroendocrine-immune axis to maintain homeostasis."[10]

You can do abdominal breathing while engaged in other activities, but practicing at rest with eyes closed will increase your awareness and knowledge for use when needed. Sit or lie and place your hand on your abdomen, on or below the navel. This may be helpful to cue breathing from that area. Begin to observe your breath for several cycles without introducing effort. Become aware of the action of the diaphragm and abdomen during air movement. The diaphragm is the thin dome shaped muscle that stretches across the bottom of your rib cage, under your lungs. When it contracts to draw in air, feel the abdomen expand under your palm to accommodate lung expansion as they fill with air. Notice how the minimal chest movement is necessary to breathe in this way. The diaphragm then relaxes and moves upward and the lungs recoil as air moves out of the lungs.

Continue breathing this way and become aware of the abdominal organs being rocked, compressed and released. Feel the expansion into the sides of your abdomen, deep into your pelvis and around toward your back massaging lymphatics and circulation. This is similar to the breathing style of a musician who plays a wind instrument or how an accomplished singer breathes. They can draw in a bigger volume of air and sustain the deliberate release of breath for extended notes by using their diaphragm. Spend several minutes experiencing and observing.

Vagal nerve stimulation and reset occurs with slow deep (diaphragmatic) breathing at a rate of about five to seven breaths per minute. This sends a message to the vagus nerve and autonomic nervous system that you are safe. You achieve the rhythm by breathing about every 10-12 seconds. Do not necessarily hold your breath, but allow the natural balancing pause between inhalation and exhalation. After breathing this way for three to five minutes, observe how you feel. Make notes about the various parts of this Heart Activity in your journal.

Healthy vagal tone has also been documented as an independent predictor of mortality in cancer by "improving prognosis" and "evidence supports a protective role... specifically in the metastatic stage."[11] The sensory and motor neurons of the vagus nerve convey information important for optimal health and onset of recovery. This can be as important for managing the environment where you work and where patients receive their treatments, including the verbiage used during diagnosis and treatment. This is a good reason to guide your patients in diaphragmatic breathing when it is possible and appropriate. It will help them create a feeling of safety and healing within an intentional healing environment. If it is influential to an outcome of disease to do so, it can likely promote a more optimal healing or preventative environment too.

Awareness and Presence

Presence has to do with your depth of awareness in a given moment or encounter. Your breath can be used to integrate physical presence with qualities that heighten your presence through conscious awareness. This is helpful when you desire to be a therapeutic presence for a patient or be more fully present in a meeting with your manager. Sincere empathy, active listening and honesty are examples of *being* in this realm.

Presence also has to do with the present moment, here and now. Time and place meet in the only moment we can truly *be* in, between the past and the future. Take note that a breath has an onset and a culmination. Each breath is, in effect, a mini lifetime. In this perspective, the totality of what *is* exists only in that present moment, life begins with inspiration [inhalation] and ends upon expiration [exhalation].

Zen Master Thich Nhat Hanh teaches, "Only this actual moment is life." To share a moment of conscious presence – a breath untainted by multitasking – with yourself or a patient is connecting, affirming, healing and priceless.

Observe within yourself the full cycle of inspiration followed by expiration for multiple breaths. For several minutes just relax and be with your breathe and *being* without judgement or specific practice. How do you feel different? What does being present feel like to you? Return to your breath. Do you notice the subtle pauses at fullness and emptiness? The action of breathing contains a sense of satisfaction within each phase. The completion of each cycle is a gift of being present. Basically, you do not even have to know when to breathe as your body's wisdom breathes for you. So allow it to happen. Do this for another minute with your awareness on any sense of satisfaction provided by both fullness and emptiness. Notice how each breath *is what it is* and how your body enters it without any anticipation. In the exhale there is no expectation. That is the fullness of the moment. In your everyday and work life, how often do you experience a sense of ease, satisfaction or completion? How can you allow for ease and satisfaction in your life? Return to your breath for guidance whenever you want allowing, receiving and releasing to be part of your *way*. Include your experience and observations in your journal.

As you relax and synchronize with the slowing breath, the satisfaction increases and the pauses can lengthen. This is a physiological balance point of neutrality and respite which facilitates oxygenation and cellular respiration. It is a balance of Yin-Yang, where emptiness leads to fullness and returns, which creates wholeness from which satisfaction arises in counterbalancing, interconnected and continuous undulating flow similar to the concept of the infinity symbol.[12]

In your job, when do you tell a patient to take a deep breath? Why do you do this? Several reasons may be: to inflate the lungs for assessment, to suggest focus or stillness, to oxygenate, distract or calm. When do you breath with a patient? It is easy to take for granted this instinctual means of connecting with another and increasing presence. The instruction to 'take a deep breath' is often a quick command. Spoken in this way, the patient responds by anxiously sucking in air often with raised shoulders, as if taking a last breath before submerging for an unknown period of time. Speaking calmly and breathing comfortably deep and slow elicits the parasympathetic nervous system and a restorative physiology. You must match the state that you want your patient to achieve, which makes you a facilitator of healing.

For a day observe yourself during different activities and environments, and notice how your breathing and presence change. What do you experience when you are on a leisurely jog compared to walking quickly to patient's call? When you are preparing to call a doctor on the phone at work, is there a difference when you are calling a friend? When charting on a computer or daydreaming? When you are talking to your manager or listening to a patient? Waking naturally or to an alarm? How does any of that differ from when you drift into sleep? Record what you observe about how changes in your breathing are related to your awareness and presence. Breathing fast, high in your chest, sighing and yawning are signs of dysregulated physiology as is present in stress, anxiety and metabolic imbalances.

During the breath awareness activities, especially with eyes closed, you may experience deep relaxation and feel slow to regain presence. Deeper more stimulating breathing may alert you because it oxygenates and detoxifies. Drinking water is an important and refreshing way to improve mental alertness especially on the job. Also, at times during the day or during your work shift, you may feel similarly sluggish or have difficulty being present. State your name in the following sentence to yourself. "I am [*your name*] here and now." That verbal proclamation can switch on the conscious mind. Other simple ways to become more alert and present are to blink, yawn, stretch, flex and point your toes, stomp your feet, or walk around.

Awareness and Intuition

Intuition is a perception or knowing of something that is beyond the reasoning of the conscious mind. It may be extending one's awareness into what psychologist Carl Jung called the "collective unconsciousness."

Ancient wisdom says we are connected to each other and the environment. Martha Rogers, a nursing theorist, said in *The Science of Unitary Human Beings* that energy flows freely between the individual and the environment. Intuition is that part of our knowledge we may have lost as we became further separated from nature.

Experiments based on quantum principles have proven that information in the subatomic world is communicated between particles instantaneously, despite long physical distances. This means that you are connected to your patients on very subtle levels. Further, according to research by *The Institute of HeartMath,* the heart appears to receive and respond to intuitive information.[13] "[The] unconscious perception [intuition] often is evidenced by subtle changes in emotions and measurable physiological changes that can be detected throughout the body... seconds before the stimulus is actually experienced."[14]

Consider these examples, two actual occurrences of intuition. They also support that you can feel and know things before the brain or technology can detect it.

My personal experience was while working a night shift in ICU in a small community hospital. It seemed all the monitors and assessments were stable, but something just did not feel right about one patient. He was reclining with the head of his bed elevated about sixty degrees. I ordered ABGs even though he said he felt fine. The respiratory therapist said the patient looked good, and proposed he would do the ABGs after he returned from his dinner break. I successfully persuaded him to do the lab before his break on the basis that he was the only RT in the facility. The moment was surreal when I looked at the incongruent test results and then at my patient. I felt disbelief and had a tightness inside my stomach. It seemed I heard the staccato musical sound effect, like in a movie just before something scary happens, as I asked, 'Are you sure that you feel all right?' My patient's eyes rolled back and his body went limp. I initiated emergency interventions without any delay. I had detected unexplainable, progressive small changes that were immeasurable on the equipment, but that added up to his deterioration.

Another situation was the time my friend Andrea and her daughter, Carmen, were at a restaurant in Bali. They sat to have a drink and look over the menu. Something about the place did not feel right to Carmen. She looked around, noticing people, reading signs, observing their environment. The place was empty, only a few tourists. Carmen suggested they go elsewhere. She could not distract herself from her urge to leave and said she would leave on her own if they did not leave together at that moment. Andrea did not feel the urgency, but could sense Carmen's determination and unusual restlessness. They left without finishing their drinks. Carmen felt it was lucky timing for them that a transport car was available right outside. Only moments down the road, there was an explosion behind them. Smoke and debris spewed from the restaurant they had just left.

⊕ Can you entertain intuition as an important assessment skill? Have you ever walked onto your unit at work and, even though it is quiet, you sense that is has been a rough day for the prior shift? Can you sense things about your patient that may not be evident to others or detected by the technology? Can you perceive a possible need behind an issue of contention such as the need for rest or recognition when a colleague or patient is upset?

How is it that you can do this? What cues did you pick up on? Where and what did you feel in your body? Where are you reading or sensing this information from? Make notes in your journal and add to them as you increase awareness of your intuition.

Albert Einstein said, "The only real valuable thing is intuition." He believed the mind is servant to the gift of intuition. Does it seem that our society and medical culture has forgotten the gift and honors the servant? He would agree. Self-regulation skills for building coherence, especially through the heart, will facilitate increased intuition and awareness.

Integration

Awareness is a skill you will use throughout the Process and continue to improve with frequency and diversity of use in your life and relationships. As you apply the concepts from this step, what comes from this will be the foundation of the rest of the AH SUCCESS Process. With awareness, you learn where you are and get an idea where you want to go.

On a new page in your journal, write "A - Awareness" as the title at the top. Prepare yourself for this experience by doing the A-B-Cs.

Consider a specific stress(or) related to work or a situation that is keeping you awake at night. Become clearer on the issue as you breathe by shining the light of your awareness on what, where, why, how, when and who related to that stress(or). Observe your experience from the safe distance of the observer. Look at the preceding events, the stress or situation, and the circumstance and feelings that followed. After you do a review, visit different perspectives of it. Look into the layers or sequence that it is made of or that led to it.

What is going on inside of you? This is where healing begins, on the inside, within the environment of your mind and body. Become consciously aware of how you feel, what your think, what conversations echo inside. Observe your breathing for changes in speed, pattern, cadence or quality as you wonder. What do the variations indicate to you - resistance, readiness, willingness, openness, ability, doubt, acceptance? Make notes in your journal about your experience with this activity up to this point.

How does this stress or situation affect you? What trajectory are you on as a result? What do you want to be different? What are different outcomes that could have happened? Where were the opportunities and choice points? What was needed? Run through alternate scenarios and see how you are called to be or do differently. How do these differences feel to you? Continue your notes in your journal.

Notice any sensations in your body. How ready are you for things to be different? How willing are you for this to be different and for you to change? How will you know that you have success? What will success feel like?

Observe what feelings and sensations or internal dialogue change for you as you feel successful. How would your *response-ability change* if similar circumstances present again? Notice the dimensions of your awareness. When the experience feels complete for you, it is complete. Summarize your experience and observations in your journal.

CHAPTER 7

HOLD SPACE FOR POSITIVE POSSIBILITY

From where you are, your success may seem remote or even unreachable. You may be tired, depleted or full of doubt. Your gauge for the route and distance to your goal is by logic and linear measure. When creating something, as you are – change, health or a dream – there are different, natural laws that apply. Things can flank into alignment, vanish without a trace and burst into being. This is possible in part because of the unacknowledged space that logic and planning do not account for. This is a difference between planning and creating. Rigid plans eliminate options, creating is intentional by metamorphosis, remaining open to possibility. When your mind is fixed or cluttered, breathe and find the gap between the thoughts. When you're anxious and breathing too quickly, find the pause. Likewise when you perceive everything is going wrong, find the crack, and let in the light of possibility. We will venture forward to approach understanding why this is transformational.

St. Francis of Assisi, patron saint for ecologists, offers this advice, "Start by doing what's necessary, then do what's possible." He further shares, "... and suddenly you are doing the impossible." What is necessary? Worry? Fastidiousness? Complaining? Sleep? Stillness? Why is it necessary? What makes one thing possible and another impossible?

Chuck Yeager flew his plane faster than the speed of sound before it was deemed to be possible. Nik Wallenda has eleven Guinness World Records and has successfully performed many never-before-accomplished death defying feats. Mahatma Gandhi used compassion to overcome oppression and single-handedly demonstrated nonviolence as a powerful substitute for violence. You defy mathematical odds and laws of nature when you bring people back to life after a cardiac arrest.

Who decides something is impossible? How does one do the impossible?

According to Wallenda, in his recent book, *Facing Fear*, "Step out in faith, and rise above whatever is holding you back."

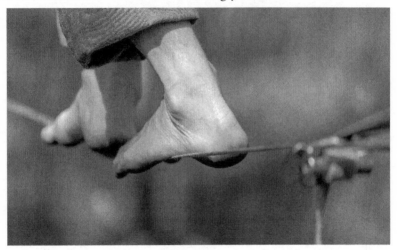

Photo licensed from Adobe Stock / rommalic

Holding space is about opening to what is possible, which means it is within this act you intentionally reach into possibility.

Logic

Logical, systematic thinking is necessary for the focused, intense activities of your job because it facilitates predictability, efficiency, and productivity. All thought is creative and drives energy to the object of its focus. The energy of intentional thought in your work environment is immense and leads to problems being solved and objectives being met within a consensual framework and toward a common goal. Efficiency arises from familiarity, repetition, patterns, and systematic ways of handling tasks and challenges. However, there are common idioms that challenge logic such as, 'the best laid plans often go astray' and 'Murphy's Law.' There are many components to success that defy logic.

Time, Stamina and Endurance

The hours and years invested in your education and career are necessary for expertise, and accumulate as a valuable measure, and merit of knowledge and experience. During this invested time, you have matured and increased your capacity of what my mom called '*stick-to-it-ness.*'[1,2] Two of its components – stamina and endurance – are necessary to meet the growing mental, physical and emotional demands of your job. Let's look at their subtle differences to gain an understanding of each as important qualities necessary for achieving what is possible.

Stamina is how long you can perform at maximum capacity. A work-shift of revolving admissions and discharges, multiple emergencies, delays in pharmacy deliveries, high acuity patients, and difficult IV (intravenous) insertions all require intense performance. When you miss a break, you must double down your effort to maintain the efficiency. Then the manager asks you to stay over a few hours because of the momentum on the unit. Before agreeing to stay, you may make a mental inventory of your bank account and bills to see if you need the money. Do you also take an inventory of the reserves in your body to determine if you have the energy and nutrition along with the mental and emotional fortitude to maintain your stamina for the extension of your shift?

Endurance is how long you can perform without a specific measure of capacity. To sustain the longevity of your career, you may get massages, modify tasks to avoid repetitive strain, educate yourself and practice ergonomic awareness, take periodic vacations, exercise and try to take your breaks. At another point you may decrease your work hours or change jobs to one with less physical demands and less work-related stress.

Despite all this, some say their twenty years in nursing was a blink in time while others say their first five were difficult to endure. After multiple years of saying I was going to live in the Caribbean, while there on vacation I made a decree that I would move there within the next five years though I had no idea how it would come to be. From that moment the *way* started organizing and I accomplished the move in less than two years. The necessity of time in healing and manifestation is relative.

Self Regulation

Your employer demands stamina and benefits from your endurance, but you must become the manager of your energy and health. Changes in your energy level take place during a heated confrontation, work shifts with high patient acuities and emergencies, and over the years of your career and life. Each of us, in our own time, has to accept what Toby Keith sings, "I ain't as good as I once was, but I'm as good once as I ever was."[3] The maximum performance of stamina naturally ebbs and flows, available as needed throughout a work-shift, but will burn out quickly when persistent. The sustained moderate output of endurance will get you through a shift or a career. It keeps you going, even into the resistance phase of Selye's General Adaptation Syndrome, discussed in Chapter 4, but will also dwindle into exhaustion if not relieved.

Often nurses do not have time or energy to enjoy their personal time and family activities. Employers want as much of your time and energy as they can get. If you want some left for yourself, self regulation is necessary. As you become more resilient, balanced, and value your health, the model you live from will change and the one you work in will be affected. When it comes to realizing a dream or accomplishing success, the more you believe it, the more you become it, and the more certain you will live it.

Cycles

The cycle of shift-work spins the daily schedule of life for most nurses and hospital workers. Scheduling vacation time-off and holiday coverage is rotated between staff, while benefits accrue on cyclical measures. But these cycles do not serve to rejuvenate or revitalize the worker. They are more like the wheels that keep the productivity rolling.

Everything in nature has a cycle – ebb and flow, wax and wane, peak and trough, action and rest – as you discovered while observing your breath cycle in an earlier chapter. These natural cycles balance opposites and promote wholeness and health. Do you recognize, the Yin-Yang of these cycles?

Healing, a parasympathetic dominant state, takes a back seat to any sympathetic innervation such as the neurophysiology that occurs during a typical stressful work-shift. The way to find relief from the mental pressure, over stimulation, and energy demands in your job is through stillness, nature, healthy cycles, and creativity. A key to longevity in your career is to cultivate the mental, emotional, and physiological ability to heal and be whole.

> What can you do to balance the opposing forces involved in work-stress and maintaining health? Consider conscious activities of expression and rest, reach and recoil, stretch and balance, contract and release. These skills comprise resilience.
>
> What cycles are dysfunctional for you? By looking at them honestly, you may understand some of the *why's* and *how's* in your life such as: *Why did I get high blood pressure? How did I get stuck in this relationship or job?* What can you do to balance and create healthy cycles? Explore these questions and list the possibilities in your journal.

Openness

The skill of holding space is one that facilitates doing what is possible through openness. This may seem paradoxical because holding usually implies grasping. Often to achieve what is necessary – efficiency, productivity, competition – it is necessary to tighten up. To make what is unlikely or impossible seem possible, such as heal, compromise, or create options, openness and space must be created first. Holding space is done through release, to allow room for possibility in an otherwise closed, immovable, non-pliable circumstance. Openness, as a characteristic, requires flexible inclusive cognition, and creativity. In fact, research links openness with perceptual processing and intellect, curiosity, creativity, and the motivation to explore and engage with possibilities.

You have naturally done this before, this holding space, even if unknowingly. It is how you move forward or accomplish things. It may have occurred automatically during high motivation or perhaps with some effort such as in a negotiation. Should you find it difficult at any moment, practice self-awareness around holding space and cultivate your conscious mind toward openness. This will probably be a continual skill-polishing process because situations will challenge you in different ways. Your breath is a readily available indicator and modulator of openness.

How are you feeling right now? Are you comfortable? Muscles tight? Mind confused? Challenged with any concepts? Do the A-B-Cs. Watch your breath. Deepen it using your diaphragm and without any extra effort. Continue breathing as you begin to notice the easing, softening, opening, and stillness that occurs. Feel the spaciousness. You have relaxed your mind, and released the tension and tightness of holding into it. However subtle, this is how and where possibility can enter.

Who's in Charge?

A mind that is closed cannot grasp new concepts or possibilities, and will leave you stuck, unable to grow, even feeling lifeless. Frank Zappa says, "A mind is like a parachute. It doesn't work if it is not open."[4] A parachute that won't open cannot grasp the air to save your life. A closed mind, like a parachute that won't open, can lead to disaster. We don't mean to have a closed mind but are socialized to identify with certain performance and standards, answering to a given name or role, and playing by the norms of family, society and work. We are also deeply influenced by what is subconscious and a primitive system of protection to fight, flee or freeze.

How does a mind close when thought is spontaneous and prolific energy? Thoughts, limitations, rules, and beliefs are a major part of the repetitious loops of emotions, problems, judgements, conflicts, anxieties, and beliefs that fill your mind and can create 'mind static' on conscious and subconscious levels. These create a trap of habitual patterns in thinking, closing a mind toward entertaining alternatives.

Irving Berlin said, "Life is 10 percent what you make it, and 90 percent how you take it."[5] Traits of your personality can uniquely affect the way you perceive reality and what is possible or impossible. How you take life is likely because of your subconscious programs, which you are usually unaware of. These were mostly 'recorded' when you were a suggestible young child prior to the age of six. Hence our hang-ups, often difficult to identify and abolish, usually expose an immaturity or naiveté.

When you are learning or making decisions at work, your knowledgeable and logical conscious mind performs. It knows the rules and reasoning. The subconscious mind records information during suggestible situations and plays back the information gleaned from experience. Though it has much greater capacity than the conscious mind, it does not independently think or reason. It usually operates without your awareness, but via cues from your conscious mind to retrieve stored information for carrying out familiar tasks, or to help recognize or verify things from pre-existing knowledge, beliefs and judgements. Its library of habituated information plays like programs that pattern [control] your thoughts and behaviors into how you unconsciously think and function, which becomes your familiar persona.[6]

Imagine yourself as a 4-year-old reacting to a complex interpersonal situation involving a patient and family that you might handle in your job. What skills do you have available? At age four, you can yell, pout, stomp your feet, cry and run away. These are typical reactive responses when you are not mindful, lack skills for self regulation or get frustrated from feeling out of control. As an adult, the expectation is that you have skills to override responding with a tantrum and that you will do so. Even so, both valid and invalid internal tension and beliefs may color your attitude and how you respond, even in resistance to changing them. Finding a means to identify, express, release, or reconcile these programs and tensions is necessary for your health.

The 'observer-you' dwells within your being and watching in your conscious mind. It is aware of the subconscious writhing 'little child' inside of you who is over-tired, sleep deprived and wants out of the pressures during an insanely busy shift. With practice and training, it can also notice your inner programming driving the self-defeating behavior. The conscious mind may be open to new ideas or reject alternatives, often influenced by the trove of information stored in your subconscious that it must tame.

This stored information is not just from the philosophies recorded when you were very young. There are other circumstances where new programming enters this space, when you are in a suggestible state – vulnerable, threatened or under the influence of a perceived authority. The subconscious is where the voices of parents, siblings, teachers, managers, colleagues, doctors, clergy, lovers, and others enter and live.

For instance, you may recall the critical words of a peer, an angry parent or a harassing manager rising from your subconscious when you are stressed, fatigued or in doubt. Their negative feedback to you, especially when repetitive, can have the effect of making the negativity or criticism seem to have some truth. Whatever the challenge or authority this person seems to hold in your life or relationship, bypasses the censor in your brain and your subconscious records it. In fact, once it is in your subconscious, the background repetition of this programming can unknowingly derail your results until you consciously intervene. Some say, "Insanity is doing the same thing repeatedly and expecting different results."[7] We are usually unaware of our repetitive and reactive behaviors, and programming that do not serve our best interests. This is like having a blind spot. The subconscious is often where the seeds of this insanity and uncertainty have rooted.

Who is in charge of your decisions, impulses, the way you respond, your receptivity to new possibilities, and your secret insecurities or esteems? Is it your emotions, your mom, your big brother, a boss or the bully on the playground? Or is it your higher self, inner wisdom and knowledge?

For this Heart Activity, plan for five columns covering a two-page spread in your journal. Make the first column on the left the widest. The other columns can be narrower for small phrases or single word answers. ⓘ

List any automatic thoughts, beliefs and habits in the first column, allowing several lines to write them all down. These should include any distinctive and obscure practices, beliefs or philosophies you have or have acquired. For instance, "I have to eat everything on my plate" or "We never get to take a break" or "For it to get done right, I have to do it myself" or "I always have to be the strong one" or "I always get the heavy work assignment." It would be meaningful to include in this activity the same stress(or) you chose to work with. Include items that might be considered either 'positive' or 'negative' thoughts, beliefs and habits.

In the second column, write who said this if you can recall or how you came to believe this...perhaps from parents, relatives, a boss, a TV show, the news, a church, a classmate or a conclusion you made. To the right of each, in the third column, write the corresponding age when you can recall that influence. If you do not have any of these thoughts attributed to yourself, consider adding some that are your very own creations.

Fill in the fourth column by answering whether you still live by this.

In the fifth column, answer the question, "Does this serve me well or not?" This may take time to contemplate. Answers of yes, no, or a question mark are sufficient. You may want to journal about each separately to review the benefits and challenges they provide for you.

Finally, contemplate *who* is in charge and *whose* voice are you still listening to? Has it become an inner voice of doubt or confidence, the voice of fear or love, or is it the voice of your inner wisdom?

> What new awareness did you gain about your patterns of thoughts and beliefs, their source, or how they restrain or otherwise influence you? Turn to a new page and write about your new awareness. If you wish to change any of these patterns, write an alternate that serves you better and may enhance holding the space for positive possibility.

You know you are experiencing stress and must become aware of any causative programming and associated perceptions or thought in order to release yourself from it, thus creating space. Some good news is that it is possible to facilitate the connection between the conscious and subconscious. This is where the skills of self-awareness, observation and meditation become very helpful. It is possible to consciously direct your inner self-talk and enter new desirable programming into this space. You can accomplish this with self-awareness and conscious positive action. You must be in charge and, when you are, you can hold space and be open to new possibilities. This is where you must aim. Go forward with what you *want* rather than repeating un-serving patterns. It is empowering to entertain the many choices that present from the possibilities. When you align them with what you desire, you find suddenly you're doing the impossible.

Holding Space

You become a conduit for possibility by holding space as a way of *being* that is allowing and open. We suspend judgement in this internal realm. This is another skill sharpened by practice, necessary because our primitive programming is about detecting danger and hence reactive and protective – holding in a way of tightness. Also socially, Western culture conditions us toward labeling and looking for the negative. You must evoke a sense of wonder to be open. To do this, it may be helpful to imagine a question mark over your head as you look about in wonder and discovery, rather than having a 'been-there-done-that' judgemental approach. Why pass up viewing the sunset just because you have seen one before? With this attitude, you deprive yourself of possibility. While learning, be gentle with yourself and others. It is easy to *mis-take* an opportunity for a re-take or a new-take on things.

> 🌀 Practice having wonder, to help with holding space. Walk around the familiar turf of your home and imagine feeling curious about everything, like seeing it for the first time. Take your time doing this. Hold the space for seeing things differently. To enhance experiencing things differently, assume an obvious alternate perspective such as that of a person who is shorter than you, or look at the area as if you were an artist, a realtor, building inspector or toddler. Make notes about how being in wonder feels to you. What did you discover? Also, for your awareness, note any resistance or naysayer voices that try to speak against your success and add them to the "Who's in charge" chart you created in the last Heart Activity.

Recall an experience of stress on your job involving a patient. Maybe they yelled, were demanding, and there seemed to be no way to please them. You may have been at a loss for words, felt unappreciated or trampled on verbally. Sometimes there is nothing you can say or do. You may notice that you hold your lips tight to avoid saying anything, your shoulders and scalp could be tight, your stomach may feel gripped and your breath held.

Instead of shrinking or closing down in a standoff, release. Holding space is a way of creating openness in a tight, closed, uncomfortable or no-win situation. Another secret to holding space is once you release and create openness for possibility, the holding is done in the buoyancy of your consciousness...by will rather than might. What are the possibilities in this circumstance? For instance, a patient may have been in a state of overwhelm with their diagnosis, treatment, side effects or loss of their quality of life, and there is nothing that could mend it or no words to say. When words fail or would potentially make things worse, it is helpful to *hold space* for yourself and your patients, for positive possibilities, for emotions to settle, or for a re-connection between your patient and their sense of self.

(♡) Can you feel how holding space and a sense of compassionate wonder would support openness in the above situation?
Make notes describing what it feels like inside of you to
hold space for another.

How would doing the A-B-Cs help you hold space for positive possibility? Let's look at the A-B-Cs and how they can help. First, you become *aware* and step back emotionally – and physically if needed – from
the situation to give the person space to vent, and for you to feel safe
and observe. Second, *breathe* slow deep breaths and notice the momentary pause between the end of exhalation and the beginning of inhalation. Use this as a point of satisfaction and respite. This will *shift* your
physiology toward relaxation. It will ease tension and clear your mind
for intentional communication. Next find your *center*, for instance, in
your heart. Breathe from that area and *feel* a caring emotion in your
heart. This soothes your being, which will influence the environment
around you and even have a subtle positive effect on your patient.

Adding the experience of a heart-based emotion to the A-B-Cs is
an additional technique that tunes your body and mind into a state of
openness, non-judgement and coherence similar to the techniques and
research by the *HeartMath Institute*.[8] No one need know that you are
doing this. The caring feeling does not have to be toward anyone in particular. *You* are regulating your physiology for your well-being. This can
help prevent an immediate meltdown during an amygdala hijack and
protect you from getting caught up in a negative attitude. With practice, holding space will require minimal time and effort. By resetting
yourself, you are allowing the space for a different outcome to occur
than the trajectory the situation had started on. Your success in holding
space will positively influence the situation and the other person.

Understanding why the A-B-Cs work will help your 'logical' brain
remember to do them until they become a natural way to respond.
The A-B-Cs can activate the vagus nerve to counteract the physiology
for the human responses of fear and stress which actually "shuts off

the body's digestion and healing ability, dampens the immune system, makes it hard to think, remember, problem solve and concentrate."[9] An intention for openness (space) is like a declaration, and is necessary for healing to take place. This modulating your nervous system is more recently referred to as healing your vagus nerve. For most people, the vagus nerve is extremely inhibited because of over stimulation of the autonomic nervous system by chronic stress. Breathing slower and deeper will stretch out the pace of thoughts. Like pre-stretching a new balloon to make it easier to inflate, the breath prepares the mind for easier expansion into a sense of wonder. Becoming centered, will help you tune toward possibility because the heart, or one's center, is able to fathom the unseen and unknown whereas the logical brain cannot. Being able to use the A-B-Cs *at will* when you need them is foundational to your long-term success.

Space

Deepak Chopra, MD, author, practitioner, and teacher of Ayurveda and meditation, encourages meditators to "experience the gap."[10] The gap is between your thoughts. This space of no thought and no intention holds pure potentiality – for positive possibility. This is where you bring your deepest and clearest intentions. This is a present moment experience that arises from silence and stillness. In the gap it is likely even your breath will be 'at pause' in momentary points of balance. It is blissful in this space. Meditation expands the gap. Interspersing the stillness between thoughts and activity is one way to build resiliency. It is depleting to be "on" constantly. Rest. Be still. Hold space.

When you can create space in your mind to balance the density of thoughts you have at work, you can find ease and heal. You are integral to the healing of others by your presence. This practice will help you build and expand the capacity of the space you can hold when thoughts and words become unnecessary. The potential capacity is infinite. The expansion is your own healing which contributes to the quality of your ability to be with another (presence) and allowing for theirs.

New Science of Possibility

Bruce Lipton, PhD, is an internationally recognized leader in bridging science and spirit, and brings the impossible into the realm of possibility. He is a stem cell biologist and author of *The Biology of Belief and Spontaneous Evolution*. He speaks on the new science of epigenetics, which literally means "above the genes." In an interview with the National Institute for the Clinical Application of Behavioral Medicine, he said, "We are not controlled by genes." Instead, our perception of and response to the world controls them. [11] So when you feel stress, its physiology affects the health of your genes and body. This is why environment can activate gene expression, resulting in the creation or cessation of healthy growth.

Dr. Lipton points out that self-empowerment is found in epigenetics because you can take part in an otherwise seemingly powerless situation. Holding space for positive possibility results in the development of new supportive neural connections. This is necessary to build an auxiliary route around the ruts of habitual and limited thinking, and assumptions. These will weaken and fade from lack of use as you reinforce the new possibility. This relates to the effects of belief in the placebo effect. [12]

In an occurrence of the placebo effect, a positive belief about something can account for 30-50% or more of a positive outcome. Because thoughts are energetic and vibrational, they can influence your physiology, emotional state and your *real-ity*. The amazing thing is the placebo effect, despite mainstream skepticism, is the benchmark for research on drug effectiveness because of its reliability. Administering a placebo, such as an inert pill or procedure, raises ethical concerns. But we are looking at the placebo *effect*, which is the power of belief or expectation merited with producing the effect, rather than the intervention itself.

Research highlights the powerful role of expectation in the placebo response. It relates to steps in the AH SUCCESS Process such as *Hold Space for Positive Possibility* and *See Yourself with Desired Results* because your expectation of the result has the force of effect. Cognition and prefrontal connectivity to other areas of the brain are necessary for [expectation and] the placebo effect to occur. People with Alzheimer's lose the ability for expectation and hence the placebo effect, measured by reduced effectiveness of analgesics.[13] Professor Ted Kaptchuk of Beth Israel Deaconess Medical Center, whose research focuses on the placebo effect, says, "The placebo effect is more than positive thinking – believing a treatment or procedure will work. It's about creating a stronger connection between the brain and body and how they work together." In a related article of his research, he points out that "a key *shift* in the emerging mechanistic understanding of placebo effects is the recognition that there is not one placebo effect but many...from psychological and neurobiological viewpoints."[14] In her independent TED Talk, Dr. Lissa Rankin says that the placebo effect offers "concrete evidence that the body holds within it innate self repair mechanisms that can make unthinkable [impossible] things happen to the body."[15]

How does the concept of the power of your beliefs and expectations mesh with your knowledge and beliefs? Practice self-awareness and observation with this inquiry and make notes about your discovery. This information may challenge you as the medical model you work in has likely not yet put these principles into active clinical practice unless you are working at a facility doing related research.

Dr. Lipton explains that the new science of *perceptions controlling life* should replace the prior science based upon genes controlling life. The sluggishness within the current paradigm toward adopting this new science may be because modern medicine has such sturdy foundations of theory and practice in the old science. The new science is "disruptive technology," which is innovative but potentially uproots established thoughts, technology and practices.[16]

In the bigger picture, this is desirable and sought after. International conferences are held for great minds to gather and challenge the current paradigms by trying to come up with disruptive technologies. Using your *inner pharmacy* – neurochemistry via self-regulation – is just that. Becoming empowered with the knowledge and skills to influence your physiology, create improved biology and health, and less stress is a disruptive technology. This is preventative and affirmative; it involves cultivating health. Prevention is much easier than intervention. Rejuvenating the art and heart of caring for health, and the empowerment of nurses is a disruptive technology. Nurses are moving forward as leaders and agents of change toward health using their wisdom.

Holding space is yin, receptive, and open for possibility to enter. It disrupts the rigid thinking which traps you in a stalemate without alternatives. Allowance counterbalances judgment. It releases tension. It evokes a sense of wonder. Things become possible when rigid boundaries relax. If you desire something for yourself like a promotion or a ticket to paradise, even a soul mate, you must be open to the possibility.

Forgiveness

Forgiveness, which often seems impossible, is possible in the space between your thoughts of judgement, blame or pain. This space is how the light of possibility gets in. Who is it for and who benefits – the forgiver or the forgiven? Whether for yourself or another, even years later, forgiveness can occur because it is *for-giving* and you can give by creating the opening for another possibility. You do not have to wait for permission or a recognized holiday. You can do it now.

The suffix "*-ness*" means a state or condition. *For-give-ness* is the state or condition you must be in to accomplish the act of giving, which may involve sharing or releasing. It is not so difficult. You know how to give. What are some qualities of your state of being when you give? Open, willing, generous? In this sense, what you give is *space* for both the acceptance that the misdeed happened and the *shift* of the judgement of the misdeed. This results in a release while possibility arises. This is a perfect re-balance of yin, yang that is healing. Forgiveness shares the release between the one who held the blame or anger, and the one held in these ways – each receive what is given.

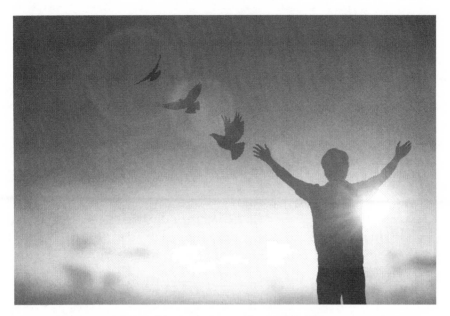

Photo licensed from Adobe Stock / Art Stock - modified by Vivo Digital Arts

Why is this healing for the one granting forgiveness? Because the psychological, neurological and immunologic affects of anger, blame, pride, guilt and shame are costly to your health. The caustic soup of those emotions bathes the cells in your body as with the physiology of stress, can lead to illness. Raising to the emotional states of acceptance and forgiveness is life enhancing and leads to restoring vitality in a profound pyschoneurophysiological way. Does this sound too fluffy? It's back by research that has proven you are measurably stronger and more capable after you have forgiven.[17]

Thomas Edison, often described as America's Greatest Inventor, said, "The doctor of the future will give no medicine but will interest his patients in the care of the human frame, in diet and in the cause and prevention of disease."[18] There are many facets of lifestyle that can support health and prevent disease, the way you think, act, eat and even how you open your heart. In this seemingly impossible way, forgiveness can help prevent *dis-ease* because it *shifts* your physiology into a life-sustaining chemistry that opens your heart and supports health and healing.

Are you are willing to do what may seem impossible and get into a state of *for-giving*? It can be for yourself or someone else. If you wish, relax and call to mind a misgiving as vividly as you can. Breathe deep and slow to move the energy held within your perspective of the situation. This is may stir emotion, just breathe through it. Evoke all the senses for information about how you experienced the situation. Spend a few moments with this to become aware of the multiple ways you are tied into this matter.

Now feel your desire to be free of carrying this burden and to be un-tethered from the associated guilt or judgement, or from being the judge. Where do you feel the desire? In your head or your heart? Let the energy of your desire propel you from the unwanted emotion into the space of possibility, toward healing. See yourself, the other, or the situation as a messenger. Ask and listen to the message. If you need to visualize it, see a parchment scroll unravel revealing information for you to read. Breathe and receive as you listen or read. Then breathe and release whatever fixed perspective, tension or emotion you are holding so you can receive the gift, the message. Feel gratitude. This does not change the past, it releases it and the future, starting the moment you release your end of the emotional rope that you hold...see it happen...whatever release you achieve is *released*. If you are having difficulty with this, bless it. This puts it in the space of grace which will reveal more to you at the right time. Allow yourself to feel the relaxation within the act of releasing and the freedom that you share with the other or the situation, because you receive as you give. Write about your experience. Trust that any measure of release will grant you relief.

Integration

From the space of awareness that you achieved in the previous step, specifically apply the additional concepts for this step as you consider your chosen stressor. Explore making room around and within the situation for ideas, alternatives and options. Be willing to open the space for new positive possibilities.

On a new page in your journal, write "H - Hold Space for Positive Possibility." Prepare yourself for this experience by doing the A-B-Cs. From the space of awareness that you achieved in the previous step, specifically consider your chosen stress(or) as you explore holding space for positive possibility.

Feel where you are with this stress(or). Find the areas of tightness, restriction, or limitation, and where it has a grip on you. Listen for meaning from what is speaking to you... your thoughts, breath, shoulders, jaw, stomach, posture, back, hands. What do they represent? Acknowledge the issues with courageous honesty. Feel your desire to see positive possibility and a different outcome with this situation, circumstance or trajectory, despite prior impossibilities.

Use your breath to create space around the stress or circumstance. Just a crack will let the light of possibility enter. What is necessary for the circumstance and ill feelings to continue? Is that what you want? Be willing to forgive and let go of what is not serving of your highest state of being. Be willing to ease up on rigidity, fear and uncertainty. If you are aware of any of these, breathe slowly from your abdomen to send calming, peaceful and safe parasympathetic signals to your nervous system. Expand your mind into the space: open, flexible, expansive possibility. Own this new spacious awareness of possibility. When you experience a sense of completion, you are done. Summarize your experience and observations in your journal.

The very act of opening and holding space for new possibility invokes its *real-ize-ation*. The concepts of *holding space* and the next step in the AH SUCCESS Process, *shifting*, work together to help you do what you previously thought to be impossible.

CHAPTER 8

SHIFT

To successfully change, things cannot remain the same. You can feel challenged even when you wish for change, because you will usually find yourself out of your safety or comfort zone in the process. Whether with your work environment, health, relationships or an experience of stress, there is a powerful component of change within your influence that is foundational. That critical piece is your state of mind. The perceived disparity between where you see yourself and where you want to be is what often leads to suffering and keeps you stuck. Change happens through *shifts*, whereas steps accomplish a journey. Some changes appear to happen suddenly while others are discreet; the action isn't clear and is often within yourself. In *Shift Happens*, author Robert Holden says this is because "you believe you live in a world when in truth the world lives in you."[1]

According to the "Banana Principle," people will choose to eat a banana instead of an orange because it is easier to peel.[2] People naturally prefer things to be easy and resist things that are difficult. People resist change because they think it is difficult. Even if the change is by choice, resistance to it will make it more difficult.

Shifting is not only within your power, it is the *way* to change. A *shift* can be tiny, but have profound effects because it facilitates overcoming the inertia that maintains the *stuck-ness* or status quo. One *shift* can lead to many, adding up to the desired overall change.

When a caterpillar follows the guidance of its inner wisdom, its DNA *shifts* expression into that of a chrysalis and then a butterfly. This metamorphosis uses the same DNA expressing differently. This is how change and transformation unfold. From *shifts* in what is, through subtle forces, as Robert Holden, PhD, says in *Shift Happens!*, mountains can move.[3]

The Sacramento River in Northern California flows over two hundred miles from its source to meet the Pacific Ocean. One would never imagine its headwaters arise from a spring gushing through a crack in the side of a mountain. Positive possibility also flows from a crack, a space in an otherwise rigid circumstance, situation or mindset. This crack is the perfect imperfection to allow for possibility, like the seed of potential in the principle of Yin-Yang.

If you cannot see options in a situation, the space you intentionally hold will invite a *shift* to occur. You do this using the A-B-Cs, awareness and breath, initially to meet what is presenting in the moment, then to observe your situation (experience of stress). Next, center to open and hold the space for shifts toward positive possibility. Allow your desire for a better outcome to draw those circumstances into being, by embodying that which you want. This act of will is a characteristic that lends one to being open. You cannot think yourself into willingness. It acts closely with choice. Both are of the creative, quantum realm, because you must first become the change you want to bring into being.

We sense space as a change in perspective, a reduction in friction, pressure or impact, a widening of vision or clarity. In doing so, energy can regain flow and move into and through that space, facilitating a *shift* of experience, perspective, options and outcomes. The *shift* can be as subtle as a release of tension that allows a breath to reset (neurochemistry) or a pause that opens new conversation in one that was in gridlock a moment prior. When you let in the light of possibility, you prepare the way for a change.

How willing are you to shift the way you see things? Look at your list of work-related stressors. Read down the list swiftly and use your first inclination to rate how willing you are to allow space for each to be different. Write your answer beside each; use zero as being not at all and five as being completely willing and open. Choosing to continue to see your stressors the same will validate your perceived circumstance, frustration, anger or suffering. But at what cost to you and your vitality? What do you gain or lose by remaining in the physiology of struggle, resistance, and stress? Answer these questions in your journal.

If you can imagine the situation or your experience as you desire, you are willing. Your willingness is a *shift* that allows possibility. Willing action is courageous because it acknowledges you are in control of your experience. Without willingness, you can be your own worst enemy. With this knowledge you can claim the power that you had within you all along, the power to choose and change.

Let Go

Willingness lies in the realm of potential. Action (*doing*) taps into this potential. The simplest action that facilitates change is exhalation. The release of breath promotes subtle *shifts,* reducing friction and resistance to change in micro-titrations, making change easier and probable. Letting go is a willing act that brings about change more dramatically, because you become what you want, released and unattached. The exhalation of breath facilitates letting go by releasing the breath and release of attachment can follow. Maybe my personal story about letting go will be helpful to you.

In my island paradise, you may find it amazing to think suffering is possible, but amidst the swaying palms and the white sand beaches, I suffered a broken heart. My island was remote and didn't have a bookstore. I rode the ferry to a slightly more cosmopolitan island to find a salve or inspiration. I bought two books – *A Course in Miracles* and *The Way of the Peaceful Warrior.*

A Course in Miracles taught that I could choose whether I want to be "right or happy."[4] I felt hurt and unhappy, but this book said I had a choice about how I feel. *The Way of the Peaceful Warrior* concurred in its teachings about suffering. Regardless of whether we get what we want, nothing external can truly heal us. Further, outcomes do not define our success, but whether we get the lesson, master ourself, and act, not react.[5] Reading these wisdoms showed me where I could get some of my personal power back.

I decided to let go of any anger and ill-feelings. I struggled with this, but I really tried hard because I wanted to be happy. To show myself how easy it was to let go, I picked up a pencil. It was the old-fashioned kind that needed sharpening... yellow painted wood with a bright blue cap eraser added to it. I held the pencil with the eraser down. I did relaxation breathing, and I focused on what I wanted to achieve. I said aloud but to myself, "Let go." Next I relaxed my fingers, and the pencil dropped. It was that easy... just be willing, relax and it will go! But to convince myself, I picked it up and did it again. It was enjoyable to let go. After a few more times, I tried it with my mind. I came up with a visualization and went to work on letting go of my hurt and anger.

What did I do wrong in my practices of letting go? This is so funny. I never noticed my mistake. I told this story repeatedly for others to learn from. After I shared it with one client, he became my teacher when he asked, "Why did you pick it up again?"

"What?"

"The pencil. You picked it back up after you had already let go!"

I laughed deeply at myself. Our exchange provided a great lesson. After you let go of something, don't pick it back up.

This is what happens when you think you've moved on and have gotten over an issue, but mentally pick it up again when triggered. Why does this happen? It's a habit and the process to change it involves awareness.

Be willing to let go, even let go of trying. For a *shift* to happen, you cannot hold on to the thought, feeling or energy of the soon to be old way. You must allow for change by holding space.

Grieving is a process of moving to acceptance. The stages are: denial, anger, bargaining, depression, acceptance. It is most commonly associated with the loss of someone through death. However, it can occur in varying measure with any loss – loss of your great grandmother's diamond necklace, leaving a relationship, changing jobs or relinquishing grip on *old ways* and habits. Over time, if it is difficult to let go, consider if and where you may be stuck in this process. You cannot hold on to the old and have the new. You cannot dwell in two different physiologies either.

> As *A Course in Miracles* asks, "Would you rather be right or happy?" This applies to an argument resistant to negotiation, an unhealthy workplace environment, or an incessant thought that perpetuates your anxiety. Consider the difference for yourself and choose one instance without regard for any specific situation. Note your choice in your journal as an empowering declaration, "I choose to be..." and fill in the blank with *right* or *happy*. Declare it quietly and aloud several times and feel our resonance with your declaration. Then say, "I AM!"

Carl Jung maintained that "what you resist not only persists, but will grow."[6] The longer you resist addressing a problem, the more difficult it becomes to do so. The longer you stay in a stressful work environment it becomes the norm and stress neurophysiology also becomes the usual, so it becomes more difficult to leave. This is in part why stress (resistance) leads to worsening symptoms over time that can become a chronic and debilitating illness, or a failed relationship or endeavor.

Imagine that you are engaged in a game of tug-a-war and there is a counter-balancing of might/power between you and your opponent. If they pull stronger, then you will ramp up your effort. They respond by increasing their resistance. Hence, you get more of what you are giving, which is resistance. If you ease up, they will too. And if you let go of your end of the rope, with no more resistance for your opponent to pull against, they will feel their own energy come back onto them and topple backward. They are left 'holding the rope'. Even if they shake it at you and tease, the choice is yours to remain released or pick up your end again. Do you see this choice a point for change?

Momentum

The intentional space you hold for possibility is available for the necessary *shifts to occur*. If you still feel things are stuck, you need momentum. *Letting go* reduces resistance. *Forgiveness* removes tethers. Doing both helps build momentum by the combined releases of energy. This transformative process converts the potential energy locked in the limiting thoughts and judgemental beliefs into kinetic energy of movement.

Choose one of those limiting things found in your chart from the 'Who's in Charge' Heart Activity in Chapter 7. Read it. Then, close your eyes and feel how your mind clings to this un-serving concept. Begin to notice the weight of carrying it and the energy it takes to grip it with your attachments. Feel yourself tire of its uselessness. Feel yourself become willing to let it go now. Exhale and feel any associations and tension from the un-serving concept leave. Completely let it go from your body and mind on exhalation. Breathe and continue to feel yourself free of it. Feel the new neurochemistry of relief and ease.

Remaining at ease, read the alternate concept you wrote. Experience it as you read if it positively resonates for you and you are willing. Imagine breathing it in. With eyes closed, allow an easy full breath, then another, allowing the *shift* to happen deeper within your being each time you inhale. Embody the new supportive concept. Now explore what is different for you with this new affirmative perspective. How do you feel? How has your breathing changed? What does your life feel like and look like now? Write key words that convey these desirable feelings and observations in your journal.

See yourself in a situation where you normally would earnestly apply that limiting strategy, but this time use the new affirmative perspective. Visualize it through to its conclusion. Be at ease in mind and body. You are already there, you have taken a different path, so stick with it. Of course, you can always pick that old way back up again. The choice is yours. Make notes in your journal.

When in resistance, if you are having difficulty letting go, ask your inner self, "What am I refusing to accept or release that, by doing so, will serve my highest state of being and greatest-good?"

Using your breath as a tool to guide your *shifts* is powerful. Thoughts follow breath. Tending to your breath directs your awareness. When you discover an answer, work with it. If you are unclear, stay with your breath and see what comes up for you. You can easily add supportive intentions such as: *Breathe in love, breathe out frustration; Breathe in peace, breathe out disharmony; or Breathe in clarity, breathe out confusion.* Following a *shift* your breathing will change, likely to more relaxed and easy.

Paradigm Shift

Paradigms unite and divide cultures, communities and families. The thoughts and beliefs you became aware of in the "Who's in Charge?" activity in Chapter 7 contribute to your personal paradigm, as does your education, experiences, and the policies and regulations of your job. It is stressful to have your paradigm challenged. What situations challenge your paradigm?

While a paradigm is foundational to your *real-ity*, health and being, it is beneficial to examine and understand your own so your can tend to it with upgrading shifts in consciousness. sA paradigm *shift* is a fundamental change of underlying assumptions that lead to a major change in thought, perception, action, values or mode of operation. *Shifts* in a paradigm often appear incremental to your reasoning mind. However, the effects are not merely linear, but rather multidimensional.

(ᗰ) Consider your personal paradigm. What do you stand for? How does your paradigm serve you in health, family, work-life balance? What paradigms do you live, work and interact with in your daily life? Where are they in agreement? Are there any parts of yours being challenged, perhaps in your work, related to your stress? For success, paradigms need commonality, not necessarily the same, but in healthy Yin-Yang relationship which require *shifts*. Spend time considering where you are being asked to *shift*. Where will you resist and where may you be willing? It is deeply empowering to understand yourself in this way.

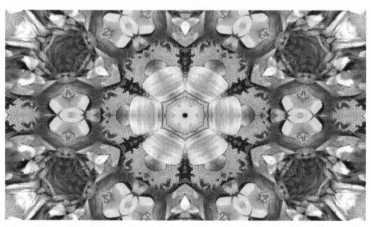

Photo licensed from AdobeStock / okanakdeniz - adapted by Vivo Digital Arts

For many years, I worked with glass as a medium for creating art. It provided many conceptual teachings. While viewing the images inside my stained glass kaleidoscopes, concepts related to *shifting* played out as I rotated the wheel. As I described the results of *shifting* within a paradigm above, the intricate prismatic effects from subtle *shifts* in the loose bits of sand, shell and glass in a scope's wheel reflect throughout the entire image. These influence other changes and produce more intricate results, just as *shifts* in perceptions and thinking can produce in your life.

According to quantum physics, everything is in motion, so things are certain to *shift*. Staying the same or stationary does not align with natural order, which is about change. What you bring to your work as you *shift* into healthy patterns, is subtle but can affect impressive *shifts* for yourself, your patients and your work environment.

Another insight I gained from my experience as a glass artist that applies to *shifting* is about balancing force and intention with timing. Glass seems fragile because it can easily shatter. It also has strength, which must be overcome in order to break or 'cut' it. An amazing thing is that in the craft, the glass isn't 'cut'. Rather, a scratch made on its surface, specifically known as a score, interrupts the structural bonds of tension in the surface of the glass. Following the score with manual firm pressure (intention) in a specific way, will direct a sequential *shifting* of bonds so that the sheet of glass will split smoothly along the score. The *feel* of this *shift* is amazing.

Shifting perspectives toward an agreeable, cooperative outcome with someone from a prior point of rigidity, provides a similar progressive release of tension and feeling of success. In both glasswork and situations on the job, timing plays a key role. In glasswork, during the time that follows a score, the 'colder' the score, the more difficult it is to split the glass, however, it will remain possible. You surely know what a missed opportunity feels like and how attempting to get it back can be difficult. However, it may not be impossible.

The illumination of a stained glass window with the varying intensity of light through the day, will provide the viewer a renewing delight as the colors dance and change. Allowing the light of possibility into a situation or mood makes things look different and can *shift* the perspective, highlight options and affect outcomes.

The effects of space, light, *shifts* and perspective often become more evident in the big picture. Gently highlight for your patients and family members, the importance of the warmth of a hug, connection through a held hand, their smile, gratitude or other visible rays of their inner-light. This is eloquently explained in this quote by Dr. Elisabeth Kubler-Ross where she compares people to a stained glass window, "... they sparkle and shine when the sun is out, but when the darkness sets in, their true beauty is revealed only if there is a light from within."[7]

Reflect and Shift

The cleaner and higher quality of the mirror inside a kaleidoscope, telescope or any optical equipment, the crisper and clearer the images. I made kaleidoscopes with optical quality mirror because it produced a less distorted image for the viewer. I also assembled them in a lint-free environment and handled them without creating fingerprints. Consider using this example as a metaphor for your paradigm and how clearly you have examined it and know yourself. Your paradigm projects into the world your perspectives, interpretations and values via your words, actions and how you treat others.

The information you take in about what you are viewing in your life is like the shapes, textures and colors that make up the items in the kaleidoscope's wheel. The image you see "out there" is a reflection of your interpretation, via your paradigm onto the world or a situation. In this way the world is not separate from you, but it exists within you. Your experiences show you what you want or need to see as a product of your paradigm, resulting in a *real-ity* that may be true for you but will differ from that of others. Isn't that amazing? We all see the world our way. Even though there is a large margin of consensual reality, variations occur because we see what we are looking for and what fits our paradigm. Your willingness to become aware through a reflective practice, is comparable to the quality and maintenance of the kaleidoscope mirror. Observing things as they truly exist are functional results of how well you come to know your mind, fears and personal paradigm, because, like a kaleidoscope, the reflection (what you see *out there*) is dependent upon the reflected (what's *within*).

The greater the distance between your awareness and your thoughts, the greater the potential distortion in to reflected image you see "out there". It is metaphorically pale, less crisp and less true. This disparity represents the potential for growth toward acceptance and understanding, using awareness. The better you know your own thoughts through meditation and self-reflection, the sharper and clearer your awareness.

Hence the sharper your image of *real-ity.*

You can practice cultivating a clear awareness and being honest with yourself using the Easy as A-B-C Technique, the AH SUCCESS Process, and meditation. When the image is again muddied, as it naturally will especially during stress, you can become aware and again observe with wonder. Then choose to hold space and allow a *shift* with something in your perception or paradigm to help clear things.

How deeply you review and release can be vast and is up to you. The intention here is for easing the immediate and long-term detrimental effects of stress for health, empowerment and influence. This is an impactful intent, but as with any tool, the results lie in the skill of its user. I encourage that you practice any moment you can, because the keys to taming the effects of stress are in taming your responses to it. Cultivate self-empowerment by increasing your capacity (resilience) for *shifting* your physiology. Follow through with aligned positive thought, choice and action to influence and improve your health, environment and situations.

Integration

Shifting is the third step to move from your stress to success. The space you hold, provides for you to now *shift* your awareness and expand into the space for new, positive possibilities.

On a new page in your journal, write "S – *Shift*" as the title at the top. Prepare yourself for this experience by doing the A-B-Cs.

Where do you sense your internal mirror? Is it different from where you sense your paradigm? A paradigm is often more heady, and one's mirror, more heart. Reflect inward about the concept of tending to your internal mirror, polishing it with a desire for clarity of direction and purity of intent. Combine this clarity with the awareness of your paradigm and cultivate an intimate life-enhancing relationship between the two. Spend a few minutes with this.

Intent is important and influential. Desire is the fire. You must be honest with yourself about both to create what you want. Be sure there is congruence between the two. If stress or a situation is bringing down your health, doing the same things will not get you different results so you must be willing to *shift*.

Consider projection of your positive possibility into the world. It is helpful to have your eyes closed to feel the potential. See with your mind, feel with your heart. Breathe and feel your readiness in your mind, body and spirit. Venture into the space and feel yourself move as you let go of anything that previously held you back. Follow your feelings into the lightness, buoyancy, openness and expansiveness. You are here... in possibility. You *shifted*! Enjoy and become deeply familiar with this realm. Dwell in possibility. When the experience feels complete for you, it is. Summarize your experience and observations in your journal.

Remember what is within you projects into your relationships, work challenges and health. If helpful, use metaphors to facilitate insight. Use the Easy as A-B-C Technique to guide and *shift* from fearful thinking to non-judgemental unconditional awareness, then observe. Take your time doing this to facilitate the next step, unlocking inner wisdom.

CHAPTER 9

UNLOCK INNER WISDOM

Trust is integral to success. Many brilliant and creative people trust their gut or use inner knowledge to guide their success.[1] Inner knowledge, self honesty and integrity, which you have been honing in the previous steps of the AH SUCCESS Process, build self trust, and unlocks your inner wisdom.

What or who do you trust? How does it feel to give trust? Where do you experience trust: in your head, your heart or gut? Who trusts you? How does it feel to be trusted? What are qualities of trustworthiness?

Review your results from the Heart Activity, "Who's in charge?" in Chapter 7. What qualities of trustworthiness do the speakers of the voices emulate? Do you trust them by way of authority, respect or choice? Do you trust yourself? When do you *not* trust yourself? In each case, how do you know? What qualities of trustworthiness do you embody?

Recall the Heart Activity in Chapter 6, "Where are you?" Is there any relationship between where you found yourself and your sense of self trust? Write your answers and explore this further in your journal so you can gain clarity on this relationship. This discernment assists with unlocking inner wisdom.

Listening

When you mindfully become more aware of your internal environment, it is not uncommon to find a circus of thoughts in your mind. It is not surprising that many are repetitious. This is a hallmark of an stressed or untrained mind. Not a mind lacking intelligence, but one that runs you, instead of the other way around. You want to choose your thoughts and responses, and listen clearly to your inner wisdom.

Stress not only contributes to having turbulent thoughts but also physiologically challenges your ability to focus and tune in to your inner wisdom. These thoughts represent ideas, impulses, questions, self-talk, and often the misguiding voices of fear, doubt and self-sabotage.

Remember, the conscious mind is creative and ego-oriented. The subconscious is a recorder of experiences and information. So while your conscious mind is producing idea, your subconscious is playing back recordings of potentially conflicting information, which may block or cause doubt about inner wisdom. Following your breath is an easy, accessible tool to guide you beyond the turbulence in your mind. It can then guide you toward discernment of trustworthy messages from your inner wisdom, which you may know as a sixth sense, intuition, insight or hunch.

Listening, as used here, is a skill of observation of using your senses to glean information for the sake of understanding. This is beyond hearing using the vibratory, conductive experienced through the body's ears. You may do this for yourself or while deeply listening to a patient. You may hear an inner voice or feel a sensation such as attraction or resistance following a thought. You may get in impression, a flash of information, or 'see' an image in your mind. Intuitive information can come to you so spontaneously that you dismiss it or attribute it to luck or coincidence.

It may take practice to convince yourself of the trustworthiness of your intuition. The idea is to seek the answer from a more reliable source than your thoughts. This is a *thrival* skill to cultivate, similar to how you learned to learn to trust your decision-making skills.[2] This idea finds support in research about nurses in coronary care revealing the imperative "...to recognize and teach the concepts related to the intuitive and precognitive components of making decisions in clinical practice."[3] Listening is one such concept.

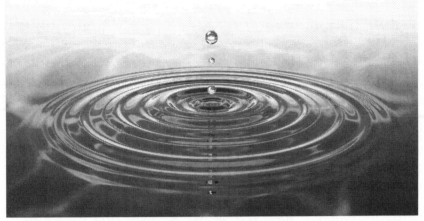

The ripples from this water droplet are a metaphor for the impact of a single thought on your quiet mind. Imagine the turbulence from the typical 30-40 thoughts per minute.[4]
Photo licensed from AdobeStock / peterschreiber.media

Meditation

Meditation can help hone your skill of listening and acquaint you with this dimension of awareness where the mind is more spacious and the thoughts are quieter than with logical reasoning. This practice will also help you become more mindful during waking activities. This is because of the quality of brain waves produced during meditation, which represent the higher energy and mental acuity associated with perception and consciousness. Researchers studied these brain waves during meditation in Tibetan Monks advanced in their meditation practice. The monks showed the highest frequency of gamma brain waves ever recorded. Researchers think theses frequencies play an essential role in nerve cell communication and demonstrate that thousands of nerve cells synchronize at extremely high speeds.[5] This synchronization is a component of the desirable optimal state of coherence.

Your brain changes by adapting to repetitive activities and thoughts by creating new neural pathways. This ability, called neuroplasticity, has dissolved the limits once imposed upon diagnoses involving neurological damage and may play a role in the brain health related to dementia prevention. This puts new emphasis on the concept of 'use it or lose it' because it also means that not exercising a brain skill will cause the corresponding area of the brain to be diminished. For instance, the hippocampus, part of the limbic system of the brain, plays an important role in long term and spatial memory that enables navigation. Relying on a GPS may have a negative effect on brain function, especially on the hippocampus, according to recent studies.[6]

> (𝒷) Consider what assessment and skill-based tasks have been replaced with technology in your job. Muse about the benefits and trade-offs and note in your journal. Most benefits were likely time saving in some way. But, note which ones removed time with the patient, such as: observation via cameras over bedside presence, automatic machines versus intimacy as in holding the arm of a patient while obtaining their blood pressure, or using a vein finder instead of tactile and intuitive skill. How do you experience stress related to technology? Record you thoughts and any frustrations you may have.

In a mindfulness meditation you observe your thoughts, while in a stillness, and any response to them. This observation is done in a state of wonder, absent of judgment or reactivity. A disturbing or negative thought can cause mental turbulence, which compounds by your reaction to it. When present-minded, you can more easily become centered and discern inner wisdom.

You can use mindfulness as a guide to behavior modification through awareness. To direct your thoughts, your reactions to them, and listen to the whispers is to find success and empowerment from self-regulation and self-determination on a sweeter, deeper, more meaningful level. This allows expression in life from your essential truth. The richness of this connection strengthens your sense of belonging, which will support everything you do and every challenge you face. It can facilitate a measure of disarmament from the threat-anticipating readiness of chronic fight-or-flight stress.

Symbolism

Symbolism is an ancient form of language understood by the subconscious mind. This language conveys information through symbols, pictures and metaphors. Metaphors are a comparison between two seemingly different things that suggests a likeness. This comparison is usually symbolic which communicates meaning on a different level than using words. Words have definitions to facilitate linear association and thinking, and are the preference of the logical brain. However, your brain can learn to understand the impressions, pictures, metaphors and symbols from your inner wisdom by association, which gives rise to meaning.

An example is how the interpretation of a dry throat during stress guides the intervention. A doctor may tell you to stop breathing through your mouth, drink more water, and prescribe some medication. These symptom-based interventions may palliate them. It is further possible to interpret the symptoms with insight from your inner wisdom. Perhaps you are not being able to speak up or a relationship is strangling your creativity. Maybe you feel you are choking in your job or cannot cough up what you want to say. Looking at symptoms and situations metaphorically can be very helpful with gleaning meanings and messages from *ill-ness* or *dis-ease* via your inner wisdom.

The work of Louise Hay was an early influence for me in considering the potential root causes of physical illness. Illness may contain metaphors that are clues for healing, as I found when I had autoimmune-thyroid symptoms. The concept, state and process of healing can be filled with metaphors, some common and others unique to the person experiencing it.

Louise Hay suggests that adrenal symptoms can result from the glandular effects of the lack of self-care, prolonged anxiety, or chronic feelings of defeat. Do you experience anything similar in relation to your job stress? Stress burdens the adrenal glands resulting in a feeling of fatigue on a deep level It even weakens your immune system, especially when stress is prolonged. Perhaps this example seems obvious to you. Inner wisdom can be so clear that your brain can make sense of it. Often, however, it will go unnoticed or seem illogical, which makes it no less valid. You must seek to relate or connect the information intuitively.

Consistently improve your ability to listen to this internal feedback system, consider the meanings and messages, develop trust, and use it guide your choices and decisions.

> ⊗ What sensations and messages do you get in your body? How responsive are you to them? Do you commonly dismiss or listen to them? How does the situation or environment affect your attention to the messages? What can you do to improve your responsiveness to the communication attempts from your body? Mindfully attend to them as you inquire: What's eating at you? What is smothering you or breaking your heart?
>
> Ignored, the signals may get louder and with more serious effects, possibly progressing to an ulcer, or heart attack-like symptoms. Explore your answer to these questions in your journal.

The metaphors and examples above could seem loosely associated because the meaning and impact of messages can be unique and personal. The following example may provide a more graphic picture that most stress-challenged nurses could relate to.

There is a condition, according to an article in report *Harvard Health*, that "almost exclusively affects women" and is stress-induced. This thought to be an easily overlooked condition is Takotsubo cardiomyopathy or broken-heart syndrome. The major symptoms are chest pain and shortness of breath, "indistinguishable from those of a heart attack." It is a weakening of the ventricle wall and ballooning of the ventricle chamber into a shape that "looks like a tako-tsubo: a round-bottomed, narrow-necked vessel." Its precise etiology is unknown but seems to be "the result of severe emotional or physical stress," possibly from "sudden surges of stress hormones like adrenaline."[7]

It is amazing that the heart can actually change shape and resemble this Japanese vessel used for trapping octopuses. Can you conceptualize that metaphor? The heart is acting as a container, trapping strong emotional energy to prevent overwhelm from severe stress. I encourage you to look it up online to see the astonishing photos and more information.

Colleen, a worker's compensation nurse, experienced increasing, unresolved stress for several years because of a disability which occurred in a hostile workplace environment and precipitated a career change. Besides a few medications to support her heart and blood pressure, the major focus of the treatment was reducing and resolving stress, rest, and recuperation. Fortunately, she, like most people, recovered rapidly with no apparent long-term heart damage. A glaring message from this condition is that stress is *at the heart* of the matter. Colleen's words of wisdom gleaned and shared were, "It's not worth it to have the stress of a job that involves an unhealthy environment because your health is more important." Sustainable success, empowerment and influence start and are maintained with self care.

> Go deep within and listen to the whispers. At the soul of your being, seek your truth. What will serve and what is not serving your highest state of being? Go into the space between your thoughts, your heart or other *center* you connect with. Ask your deep self your burning questions.
>
> Here are a few prompts that may help you get started. What stresses you the most about your job? What is the emotion blocking your success? Do you believe you can or *can not* achieve your goals in your current position? How confident are you that you are a compassionate and competent nurse? In what ways are you affected by your colleagues, manager, patients, doctors, technology, repetitive tasks, an emergency, disorganization? What is the highest way for you to use your nursing and medical knowledge? What do you need to balance the stress you are experiencing? What are you afraid of? What are you most uncertain

of? What is in your way? When you ask these questions inside your being, you may get very different, likely more personally valuable answers, than those from your noisy, chattering mind. Add notes to your journal about what you learn.

Personal Power

Courageous patients and clients have shared with me that wisdom from their self-awareness builds confidence and personal power. They learn to trust and support the intelligence in their body to heal Following up on symptoms with inner-inquiry can lead to deep insight. This can release blocked energy that may lead to a decrease in pain, anxiety, or other symptoms.

I have also received feedback that learning to listen and trust their inner wisdom is a way of living more authentically. Referring inward for guidance and answers rather than solely relying on outward feedback, can lead to more satisfaction, clarity, better communication, more tolerance, creativity, happiness and personal power.

"I'm going to live here one day." My friend recounted my words to me while I was living in the Caribbean, years after having said them. I didn't recall saying those words, and it fascinated me I had spoken such a truth aloud. I asked my friend what he said in response. He replied, "Nothing. You said it with complete certainty." It was on that sailing vacation that the ship sailed to the place that I intuitively recognized as my *picture* of paradise. I felt its affirming familiarity within my being. Within a few years, I moved there. Following your inner wisdom builds personal power. This is the empowerment that you seek.

Intuition

Does it surprise you that intuition is a part of nursing care and caring for health?

As a traveling nurse, I worked the night shift at a small community hospital. The staffing was sparse and the nurse leadership minimally qualified for emergent clinical situations. The doctors were very traditional and conservative. For twelve hours, a licensed vocational nurse (LVN), a respiratory therapist (RT) and myself maintained the twelve-bed intensive and cardiac care unit. I was *the* critical care nurse in the hospital. Besides managing my unit, I led, or more accurately comprised the emergency code team because the emergency room (ER) physician was often delayed.[8] I also had to assess any patient before a floor nurse could call a physician. The census in my unit could increase from three to seven patients in as little as 90 minutes.

The three of us became an amazing team. Each paid attention to our patients on deep levels and communicated effectively with each other. We grew in trust and confidence with each other's intuition. The LVN did the bedside care while I did assessments and administered medications. When she called my name, going slowly from a low pitch to a higher one, I would dash. When I called the RT stat[9] for ABGs (arterial blood gasses) and instructed him to prepare to intubate, he knew not to pause.

When I completed my seven-month contract there, they told me that "the mortality rate decreased while I was there." We were such a skeleton crew we had to anticipate outcomes to provide safe care. We would not wait for a patient to crash,[10] we worked to prevent it. If only the doctors responded similarly, often slow to answer pages and sluggish to give orders. Prevention did not seem to fit into their practice paradigm. Maybe medical practice cannot be based upon nurses' intuition. The reality is that fine nursing practice often is.

Nursing intuition is an ancient yin force not unlike the knowledge used by the Amazon Shuar women to guide the planting and hunting in their community. *The field* that connects all things responds to the energy and information each of us contribute with our thoughts, feelings and emotions. We receive information from *the field* via the whispers of our intuition. Best practices in medicine are for safe, validated treatments when prescribing and administering a medication or procedure. Completely ignoring the intuition of a nurse or patient could be a problem. This is akin to precisely what the Shuar chiefs gleaned was missing in our modern society when they saw the sparseness of nature in our communities. It was evidence of our disconnection.

Nurses' wisdom is a collective of information about health and the responses of humans to life from centuries of witnessing people amidst their passages and traditions, states of health and emotion, relationships and reconciliations. It is connected to women's intuition and a mother's intuition and may have been dismissed along with wives' tales and home remedies in the past. But the wisdom women and nurses have is rich. When a nurse is at the bedside for eight to sixteen hours observing, listening, and sensing a patient's energy *shifts,* this exemplifies an inner technology to be respected. I invite you to cultivate your intuition and connection to your inner wisdom. This is another boost toward your self-empowerment.

Thoughts vs. Inner Wisdom

Inner wisdom differs from thoughts and the voice of the ego as it comes from a higher source and it reveals deeper information. It can be an immediate feeling or can arise softly and quietly. It is of light and love and never of harm. It can be direct and urgent, but it will be clear without confusing details and explanation. Conversely, the ego will argue and make confusion. The ego judges, distracts, procrastinates and can leave you feeling uncertain or regretful. Intuitive guidance will nudge or nag as a way of directing you toward something. Even if it seems illogical, there is likely a rightness about it that draws you to pay attention.

Integration

The virtues of value, integrity and discernment are necessary to glean wisdom of your true nature. As Juvenal said in *The Sixteen Satires,* "Never does Nature say one thing and Wisdom another." Inner wisdom comes from within yet connects you to universal intelligence through resonance via *the field*. Inner wisdom is holistic by its nature. You find this wisdom between your thoughts, in messages from your body, and truths from your soul.

On a new page in your journal, write "U – Unlock Your Inner Wisdom" as the title at the top. Prepare yourself for this experience by doing the A-B-Cs.

Allow your breath to guide your awareness to the spacious realm of possibility and tune in to your inner guidance. Explore it with wonder. This space is where you want to introduce only dream-inspired and success-oriented energy and thought. While centered, ask meaningful questions as you would ask of a mentor or sage to help guide you with you stress or issue. With practice you will find your process of deep self-inquiry . Watch any thoughts, recognizing and promptly releasing the ones you recognize as fear or as the imposed values of someone else. Notice how it arise for you? Most important, notice how it feels. Is it light or heavy? Do you release or constrict? Do you feel uplifted or suppressed, drawn toward or repelled? You are tuning in to what feels quietly certain within. This is a sacred relationship to cultivate.

If you are having a tough time discerning from within, yield to the flip of a coin a few times for help.

Pre-assign values to each side of the coin, such as 'yes' for heads and 'no' for tails, or heads means commit to the extra shift and tails means keep your day off to get a massage. Ask your question and do the flip.

Notice the feeling of anticipation prior and then the

immediate sensation in reaction to the coin flip. Does it constrict and repel, or relax and open? This is a clue to the 'voice' used by your inner wisdom to communicate. Also practice noticing these energetic qualities within yourself throughout your day so you will get to know and trust your inner cues.

What does your inner wisdom reveal? Any insights for going forward toward your success? When this experience feels complete for you, it is. Summarize it and related observations in your journal.

Find, know, and trust your inner wisdom from which your influence will powerfully rise. Information from within may apply globally, but is a guide for you to act locally for positive change from the inside out. Your ability to access this inner source of information and inspiration will – especially when amidst stress and stressful environments – improve by honing your skills of centering in the next step of the AH SUCCESS Process.

CHAPTER 10

CENTER

Knowing your center and how to get centered are important self-regulation skills for well-being. In this chapter, We will explore some qualities and characteristics of one's center to increase your familiarity. However, the best way to understand your center is by spending time with it. Jon Kabat-Zinn, Author of *Full Catastrophe Living*, compares being centered to feeling like you are home no matter where you are or what you must face.[1] The Easy as A-B-C Technique guides you to your center. C-Center is the middle step in the AH SUCCESS Process because it is a philosophical and metaphysical central point for your embodied awareness. It facilitates your moving forward on your journey through the Process and states of manifestation toward success. It is both quiet and wisdom-filled, a respite and a springboard. Your center is a balance point of Yin and Yang. There is a sense of harmony and wholeness found when centered.

Follow the steps for centering using the A-B-Cs. Notice your breath, observe as it slows and deepens, *shift* and let it bring you into your center. Do this with your eyes closed for now. As you become more familiar with your center. You will want to become able to regulate your energy and attention with eyes open and on the go, too. Make notes or prompts for yourself about your center and being centered in your journal. What does it feel like? How is it different with your eyes open and closed? Does your center ever seem to be in different places? How do the locations feel different or the same? See if you can get close enough to each to find which serves you most clearly and find your true center.

Be gentle with yourself. It takes practice to *re-member and re-connect* with your center in your body, life, job and world of items competing for your attention and energy.

There's a story of a villager asking a monk, "What do you do in the monastery all day, every day?" The monk replied, "We get up. We fall down. We get up..."

In our modern world, we do not stay in retreat like a monk. We have to meet the diverse challenges of our relationships, life, and job while being alert and balanced. Your job is the perfect place to practice, moment to moment, and daily. This is how your life and job can be a walking practice because it is less about you falling and more about you getting back up. Then it becomes about balance, which can be guided by cultivating a connection with your center. Let's familiarize more deeply with some of the qualities of your center and how it is used for success.

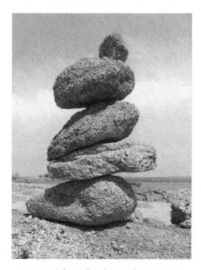

Photo by the author.

Values and Virtues

An important internal journey to embark upon is to consider your values and virtues. Values are standards or principles important to you, but are not necessarily based upon morality. Virtues are more universally accepted to be of high moral quality. You can likely come up with some values instantly, such as holidays with family, time spent in nature, eating organic food, education, providing a good lifestyle for your children, accurately administering medications, health, safety, choice, privacy.

You may note that organizations like your employer generally have written organizational values like teamwork, innovation and quality. These should also be important to you since they hire you to uphold them. If you cannot list a few of them, look them up and take them into consideration and intentionally apply them during your workday.

Discovering your virtues will help you understand your center more clearly. It may take a deeper contemplation to recognize what virtues you live by in all circumstances and at any cost. These qualities of divine measure support true happiness, and when breached, undermine it. These are qualities such as integrity, compassion, caring, gratitude and purposefulness. When your actions or those of another create a physical or emotional wound, you experience that awful feeling of loss or deception, because the expression of a virtue has been compromised. The pain can be deep, feeling as if it's in the center of your being, and it's difficult to simply shake it off. Virtue-based actions are necessary to relieve or reconcile such a moral injury. Virtues have resonance with love, honor, gratitude and care

Values add desirable attributes to your life and *get you through* challenges. Virtues are how you express life and how *you get through* it.

When you raise your resonant vibration to heart-centered virtuous qualities, your thoughts, feelings, emotions, nervous system and cells become unified and coherent. This state of coherence influences your choices and conditions your actions. Your health, relationships, work and life become energized and synchronized. It becomes possible for you to *shift* toward whatever you desire.

This is also why it is important for you, as a nurse, to have healthy, self-regulation and care skills. It relates to why you are feeling strained in a work environment that is so externally complex and chaotic. You are trying to do heart-based virtuous work in a progressively more draining and fatiguing technology-based and mechanistically driven environment. Self-preservation is necessary on a primal level when the environment keeps you in fight-or-flight mode.

Worldwide research with diverse cultures by *The Virtues Project* w discovered virtues to be universal.[2] The language of care and compassion is easily understood by your body as health-supporting and understood by your patients no matter their culture, creed or state of health. I invite you to connect with your values and virtues as a way to acquaint with your center.

Write in your journal any of your values that come to mind. No doubt several will be obvious, but spend time with this so more may surface from beneath the many expectations and obligations that you live up to and fulfill daily. It may help to look at your life and what is in it to observe what is of value to you. What is prominent in your home? What do you do with your time? What do you spend money on? What are you working toward in life? What do you think about most or dream about? After you have a few written, prioritize them. Reflect upon how these contribute to your feelings of self-worth, success, accomplishment, esteem and worthiness, or lack of these.

Now make a list of virtues you value. Circle the ones you feel you express and exemplify in your thoughts, actions, interactions and relationships, including work. Put an asterisk by any you wish to cultivate in your life and work. Reflect upon how the expression (or lack) of these virtues contribute to your feelings of self-worth, success, accomplishment, esteem and worthiness.

How are values and virtues different or similar for you? How do virtues, skills, knowledge and talent relate to one another for you? Do you experience a difference between expressing one from another? Do any make you feel higher, satiated or valuable? Which, if blocked or prevented from expressing, would cause you deep disappointment, *dis-ease*, diminish your interest and joy? Which, if blocked or prevented, would motivate you to strive? Which do you hold yourself accountable for? How do you know that you have done your best? Which are vitally important to your well-being, self-expression and joy?

Beauty

In the West, beauty is a term commonly associated with external physical attributes of a person or thing that imply aesthetic value. There is much misunderstanding around stereotypical appearances associated with the concept of beauty that few truly meet. This breeds low self-esteem which can easily root in a competitive, superficial culture. This inhibits people from embracing their own beauty found in their spirit, strengths and virtues.

Zen teaches to be fully "aware of the illusory nature of material life."[3] It "has a unique aesthetic, which includes a great appreciation for moderation, asymmetry, imperfection, rusticity, and naturalness."[4] How is a daisy more beautiful than a stone? Both are natural and unique. It is in the full expression of each that beauty is present.

The virtues you possess arise from your center and radiate as beauty through the expressions and actions of your mind and body. Being aware of your center helps you get to know your inner beauty and virtues that dwell there. In challenging times, look for beauty. You can do the A-B-Cs to center and bring forth a virtue. You may need the beauty of patience, silence, gratitude, fastidiousness or creativity to help endure or heal a situation.

The Zen and Native American concepts of beauty have been applied to the worst and most devastating of scenarios, including war, abuse, job loss, financial ruin or an onslaught of chronic debilitating illness.

You can apply it to your work-related stress. It takes sincere willingness to open and *shift* during suffering and stress. Doing so does not change the matter of your suffering, but may place it into a different context, perhaps by creating a *shift* in your physiology and space for a allowing a different outcome. It may speed healing and recovery, or provide insight toward resolving or releasing the matter or issue. If the matter is something that you want to change, then work it through the AH SUCCESS Process toward positive action.

Some say, "Every cloud has a silver lining." But highlighting the beauty for someone else may not be received with welcome because it is subjective and personal. Holding the space for the acknowledgement or witnessing of beauty is a safe and therapeutic space to be in with another person who needs healing. The beauty is that anything can have positive potential which communicates through either a call for or an expression of our beautiful virtues including *Love*. This inner beauty is unchanged by external circumstances because it is omnipresent.

⟨♡⟩ In what ways have you witnessed beauty in a less obvious situation or circumstances? Do the A-B-Cs and spend time in the presence of your inner beauty. Journal about your answers, observations, challenges, and experiences.

Connection

Learning to establish and reinforce connection with your center is important for self empowerment and healing. The source of the energy of your center is not necessarily solely generated within your mind or body. But there are areas in the body that are commonly sensed as an energetic centers. An example is the heart which is an important organ, but also has other important functions. In Chapter 6, I invited you to consider the heart as a place of awareness and centering, because including the general surrounding area and the electromagnetic field emanating from it, it is often used in practice as a center and guide.

To help your understand the experience of connection via your center, imagine two drops of water, puddled on a flat surface, each with tension surrounding and containing them separately. If slowly moved closer, at a certain point they will spring toward one another, merging as if magnetized, plumping into greater fullness once joined. When you connect with your center, there can be a sensation of expansion or a sense of opening or widening of scope or flow. Perhaps you might feel warmth, instant clarity, or a feeling of calm.

Connection also happens between people, with an animal, with a job or opportunity, even a dress, piece of art or gadget at the store. These connections can be experienced differently so within yourself it i important to be able to discern the differences. There was a time when science felt it had proven that everything in the universe was separate and there was no unifying force for all things. Though it seems the cultural norm is to still operate from this understanding, the exact opposite is true – all people and things are connected. Become familiar with this experience so you can create it within yourself, for guidance of choices, relationships and life.

Check in with how you are doing, then do the A-B-Cs. Once you are centered, consider how you experience the connection with your center. How do you feel differently in your mind, heart and awareness once you are centered? Do you experience an expansion or contraction within yourself? Do you feel heavy or light? How do you know when you are connected with another person? How do you know when you are connected with a meant-for-you opportunity? Is there any relationship between these and your center? Explore how knowing your center can help validate other connections. Record your experiences and understandings in your journal.

Stillness

As a quality of your center, stillness is the yin to the yang of daily life. It is a place of respite, quiet but not empty or devoid of life. Rather, it is full of life's potential.

There is a special time of day when you can connect with this stillness. It's most profound in the morning, when the natural world is rousing. But no matter your sleep schedule, it is found at the end of your sleep when you wake naturally rather than startled by an alarm clock-elicited stress response. This can be a typical workday, when the expectations, anticipation and leftover attitudes from the last shift rush to mind and get projected onto the day ahead. Amidst those automatic experiences it is easy to overlook the beautiful moment of awakening, which begs to be savored.

Become familiar with the semi-lucid phase of waking, before your thoughts and movement happen. This is an *in-between* state. Though destined to surface into wakefulness, your body still feels heavy as it has yet to be roused by the buoyancy of your consciousness. In other words, when possible, wake up slowly. Drift around in the spaciousness. You may only be able to dwell there for a matter of seconds. By lingering, you will become more familiar with some qualities of your center that help counter stress. This experience will help anchor your day in the resilience of stillness and wonder. As your conscious mind inevitably becomes more aware of the experience, you may desire to stay in bliss. Paradoxically, this grasping at the experience actually pulls you out of it. Notice this *shift* from *being* into *doing*. Observing the *feeling* of this *shift* will help you reset when needed throughout the day because you know the *shifts* and feelings you need to create to *center*.

It is important to mention, that being centered doesn't mean sleepy. It is actually associated with mental sharpness. But usually when people quiet their mind, relaxation potently occurs because of their underlying fatigue. Practice the ABCs at rest first. Then on the job, so resetting to your center will provide a state of resilient awareness amidst the storm when you are facing something overstimulating or challenging.

Clarity

Clarity is a quality of your center that can more easily arise from stillness. When I awoke in the sleeping loft of my island home, it was easy to meditate while looking to the East at the often smooth surface of the Atlantic Ocean. Its stillness provided a reflective surface for contemplation and space to find clarity.

It was amazing to me how such a beautiful, natural place was supported by the delicate balance of nature yet also destroyed by the same elements, such as a hurricane. This is true about the nature of our mind, as its focused calmness and clarity become disturbed and muddied by its own thoughts. Being able to center when stress sets off your inner call light will help you get clarity in the moment's chaos. Having clarity on the inside improves clarity of the outside.

Strength

Strength associated with your center differs from being muscular or having desirable knowledge, ability or proficiency. It is more stabilizing and foundational, and can magnify any of those characteristics. However, its source is not physical. It expresses artfully as it arises beautifully and gracefully from stillness, clarity, virtue and alignment. A demonstration of this is in the strength of a majestic and sturdy oak tree also having the ability to bend with the wind. This quality of strength exemplifies the synergism of Yin-Yang.

Similarly, you can respond to the call of duty, without becoming stressed and drained of your energy. Instead, you can remain clear amidst stressful and chaotic situations because you are centered, from which you gain strength, stability and insight.

Grounded

Being grounded is an intentional state that supports being connected to and energized by your center while deeply rooted in presence and resilience. Again, like the oak, physically you have a sturdy footing, as if anchored into the Earth by stabilizing roots, while having a balanced, energized stance for flexibility and agility.

Grounding, like Earthing mentioned in Chapter 3, is a concept that commonly relates to the movement of a charge of electricity toward discharge, which is a neutralization of its force.[5] A visual for being grounded is that your energy is focused, flowing evenly and efficiently around your calm, clear center rather than sparking and frittering like electricity from a live wire with a short or fray. Even as your energy interacts with your environment, it is an intentional act to ground and manage your energy for efficiency.

Use grounding when the tensions rise on your unit and you feel stressed. Balance participation in getting the job done amidst the potent and potentially depleting energetics of the situation to protect your own bioenergetics, physiology and biology. To facilitate this, you can shiver and shake off nervous or excess energy to prevent overloading your nervous system. Animals do this to transition efficiently from the alarm of a threatening encounter with a predator to once again grazing peacefully.

You know the situations that cause you to feel wired, frayed, overloaded or drained. Learning how to ground uses the strength and energy from your center to facilitate being present, aware and connected with your inner source of information with less distraction. Managing your energy while handling the energetics of relationships, situations and environments is empowering. Minimizing overloads and energy drains are an important part of maintaining your own health.

Do this brief grounding activity. While standing with knees soft or seated, have your feet on the floor. Become aware of your feet firmly on the ground or floor; feel secure and supported. Breathe in slow, deep, abdominal breaths to refresh and calm your mind and nervous system. Exhale deeply as if your breath descends from your chest and abdomen, down your legs and through your feet into the Earth. Feel anchored and sturdy. Continue to breathe and neutralize any frenetic or excess energy as it's discharged into the ground and leaves you feeling clear and alert.

This is an excellent technique for many situations such as when you want to remain calm amidst a high energy situation, a stressful meeting with your manager, or if you feel overwhelmed by a rush of thoughts. With practice you can tune yourself to precision so it will only take your specific command or intention for your body and nervous system to respond, center and ground in the face of adversity.

They showed this in the movie, *For the Love of the Game*, where Kevin Costner is a baseball pitcher. You, as the viewer, get to be on the mound with him. The noise, lights, and circumstances are just as he is experiencing them. Then the viewer gets into his head when he says, "Clear the mechanism."[6] All goes quiet. Mr. Costner becomes laser-focused, with only himself and the catcher in his awareness. This is grounding and centering by command.

In nursing school they taught me about therapeutic presence and active listening, about detachment and empathy. But it was in my massage program, several years into my nursing career, and through my well-being practice that I learned about energy, grounding, centering, touch and intention. As a nurse, I used both sets of skills.

Because patients depend upon you to guide them, you must be agile to maintain your bearings emotionally and intellectually. Grounding can be helpful. Emotional detachment may cause a mutual feeling of emptiness from a thinning of the connection with your patient. Patients need empathy. Skillful empathy comes from knowing yourself from the inside beyond superficial dislikes and favorites. The deeper you know yourself, from tears and fears to health and joy, the more capacity you build for empathy. In empathy, you do not attach to the fear of the situation nor the outcome. You stay in the moment with the person in your care while you are a grounded presence, with your heart center as your stronghold, and as a beacon for them to find their way.

Do you feel connected to your patients? How do you experience this connection? Do you cringed when they are uncomfortable? Describe any emotional distance you typically feel from them and explore the circumstances and reasons? What were you taught about connecting and distancing yourself professionally? How emotionally close to your patients is acceptable? Describe the connection you feel is necessary to have with them? Recall an empathetic experience you have had with a patient. Recall an experience where you received empathy. Make notes in your journal about these experiences.

Resonate

A common concern about energy is whether you may pick up bad energy from another person. The quick answer is no. However, you may feel bad after talking with a family in mourning, working a shift with intensely ill patients, hearing a person cry or witnessing a heated argument. The energy of the situation can influence you, but it will dissipate with time or a distraction, However, if the feeling lingers, it is less likely to be solely caused by the circumstance and more likely to go beyond empathy for the other. It may be challenging to grasp that what you see in a situation is actually resonating with a feeling in yourself. Any elusive pain, sorrow or wound you have is suspended in one of the states of grief or healing. When something within you relates to the vibe of a situation, it resonates such that you can sense or feel it, find it and heal it. If the energy vibe you picked up on is disturbing, you can do a tune-up and clear the resonance by doing the A-B-Cs. Shift out of the sympathetic experience and into one that is parasympathetic, relaxed and centered. If the vibe feels good to you, you may feel drawn or attracted to the experience, person or situation. It may reveal a part of you yet to be recognized, or a quality or talent being called upon for expression.

Integration

Because your center is the wellspring from a source that dwells within your body, it should now be easy to distinguish. Its resonance is a deep, clear and synchronous vibration that feels good. What flows through is universal and flows through all via the connection of all things, but expresses uniquely through you. When you resonate with the vibe of another person, situation or opportunity, you will know because the resonance within you will be warm, exciting or magnetizing. When connected to your own rhythm, you feel at home. It will feel familiar and synchronistic. It is from your center, a source from which to draw from. "As soon as a spring [your center] begins to be utilized as a source of water [energy, wisdom]-supply, it is more or less thoroughly transformed into a well."[7]

On a new page in your journal, write "C-Center" as the title at the top. Prepare yourself for this experience by doing the A-B-Cs.

Once you become centered, take note. How do you know your center? What changes have occurred with the ease of finding your center and in your familiarity with it? Within your center you can find stillness when you need calm and clarity, connection when feeling alone, beauty when perceiving only darkness, and trust when you need strength? It is the soulful domain of your values and virtues, and their meaning for you. This milieu makes it possible to alchemize information gleaned from the Heart Activity in Chapter 9 and experiences with inner wisdom. Bring your situation into this space and be with it now. Observe it. Listen. Be open and allow transmutation of the energy of the stress, confusion, futility and frustration into possibility and meaning. What is clarifying as other things recede? What is calling to you and how do you feel about it? What is sorting out for you? List the options that present and feelings of resonance in your journal. Notate any other information about your experience with this activity that you wish.

It is within your center you find well-being and from your center – your source – that you gain deep empowerment.

CHAPTER 11

CHOOSE

Awareness of your beckoning inner call light means there is something greater meant for you. Your desire to find it has already sparked its manifestation. You are ready to make a powerful *shift* out of the definition of insanity of doing the same thing, expecting different results. Applying effective self management to be proactive in everyday decisions, is where empowerment comes from, according to Stephen Covey. Your success is calling and your choice commits your will to make it so.

You make countless choices and decisions throughout each day. You may or may not notice the difference, but may recognize that they add to either your satisfaction or frustration. The mastery of making choices and decisions will save you from many trials, reduce stress and enrich your life with more authenticity. Mastery is accomplished by mastering moments, The moments are opportunities to express your unique potential through your choices, decisions and aligned actions. It is through these which empowerment arises.

Read the situations below. Determine if the situation is a choice or a decision. and indicate each with a C or D respectively.

    ___When your alarm clock goes off in the morning on a workday. Get up or not?

    ___When your gut is pulling and you are about to give a medication. Double check for errors or not?

    ___An order was written, but you did not get to talk with the doctor. You feel you have information that may be important to enhance your patient's treatment plan. Call or not?

___You brought a salad and fruit for lunch. Everyone else is ordering pizza to be delivered. Eat salad or pizza?

___A colleague broke sterile technique in a procedure. Speak up and stand in so they can re-prep or let it slide?

___Your bladder is signaling that it is about to burst and you are on shift amidst patient care. Resist or take care of yourself?

___There are pastries and doughnuts in the morning at the nurses' station. Indulge or walk away?

___ After greeting everyone else individually, your manager walks by you without a word. Reach out or not?

___You are called on your day off to work an extra shift. Accept or decline?

Were you able to tune in and tell the difference between a choice and a decision? The answers are within you. In your journal write a description of how you experience making a choice and a decision. Try to feel the experience in your physiology. Notice the tug and pull on values, ethics, preferences, standards, integrity, emotions and agreements. Comment on these things in your journal.

A decision is more of an act of balancing facts, logistics and rules, and eliminating options as you make up your mind. A choice may consider some of the same things, though it comes from free will, an opportunity or a right, and is uniquely your own. Consider again how you experience the difference between these two acts. Where does the energy come from for you to do these acts? For instance, it may come from rules, knowledge, experience or your imagination. The origins of the two words are revealing. The word "choice" is from "to perceive" and the word "decision" comes from a root meaning "cutting off."

You always have a choice about at least two things. Herein lies true self-empowerment.

1. You can choose to respond rather than react.
2. You can always choose your attitude.

Seeking empowerment comes with responsibility. Think of it this way, "*response-ability.*" This is the "*ability to respond*" which is coveted if you want empowerment. When you act from integrity, owning your ability to respond through choice or decision, you are more capable of reconciling any outcome and celebrating any reward.

How you exercise choice is integral to transforming your experience of stress and its impacts upon the your terrain of health. This is because wellness is deeply influenced by choice and will.[1,2] Even ordinary choices such as those related to the movement, fueling and nourishing of your body, use of natural or synthetic products, and a chosen occupation can affect your health and that of the environment. In his book, *The Extraordinary Power of Ordinary Things*, Larry Dossey, MD, visionary, author, and advocate for the role of the mind in health and the role of spirituality in healthcare, says that nothing could be more disastrous from a health point of view, than to think that our decisions, choices, behaviors and consciousness do not make a difference.[3]

Value Based Living

In the early 1990s, I developed and used my Conscious Living Education process as the basis for the well-being consultation I did with individuals. Values clarification was one of the early steps. Values provide a center from which to choose and act.

Write in your journal ten values and virtues you hold important. You might refer back to those you listed in a Heart Activity in Chapter 10. In this activity the distinction between the two is not important, only that they are of value or denote importance, worth or usefulness to you. Examples from my list are health, grace, integrity and nature.

Next, contemplate the meaning of each of the values and virtues you listed and make notes about why you they are important to you. Then write a new list and place them in priority order. The intent is to make decisions and choices from your values – which can be a virtuous quality – honoring what is important for you. Empowerment lies in your choices so as you will have less regret, self sabotage, or being influenced by external pressures.

For instance, if you truly value communication, you will have more tolerance at work with a colleague's situation because you want to understand the problem rather than merely win the argument. Likewise, if health is a value, it is easier to pass up a donut by choice. You have a good feeling because of your choice and not a short-lived sugar rush that has challenging effects on your health and immune system. If you choose to have a doughnut, make every bite a celebration, and eat it mindfully, not mindlessly or on the run. Maybe using the imagery from the experience will feed you during your next temptation, and you'll choose differently.

Power of Words

The first agreement in *The Four Agreements* by Don Miguel Ruiz, is, "Be impeccable with your word."[4] The words you use are important. As extensions of your thoughts, both conscious and subconscious, they are vibratory impulses of energy that have creative influence. What you tell yourself, especially subconsciously when you are not really listening, impacts your decisions, choices, and health.

Visualize each of these statements. "My head is going to explode I'm so tired" and "I can't think, my brain is fried." Which one do you really want to create? Even in jest, subtle jabs at your esteem can erode self-confidence and can mess with your intentions. It is less toxic to your self-esteem and more positively affirmative to say, "I'll be more clear about my decision after a good night of sleep." Do you feel the difference? Think of a couple of your common or recent stress-affirming remarks you may have made: "Work is nothing but a pain in my back." Transform them into statements of truth that are also aligned with what you truly choose to create: "I choose find a new job that is less strenuous and pays me two dollars more an hour." Write these affirmations in your journal to practice and to inspire future positive statements.

To truly *will* something to be is to make it so in the present moment. When you speak, your intentions affirm what you want. Making a choice based upon what you don't want is backwards to the mind. This involves the Law of Attraction which basically states that what you think about, you bring toward yourself.[5]

The denial hinted at by "don't" or "won't" produces inhibitory neurochemistry in your body, but has little influence on the attractive force in your mind because it *hears* in the affirmative. For instance, have you ever told a child to stop running? Did they? Perhaps they did when told, "Walk." They are more likely to respond as intended with an affirmative statement. Their brain processes the concept, as if it were a command – either run or walk. Fundamentally, the adult subconscious mind continues to work the same way. Speak truth to yourself. Say what you want and *will* it. Be affirmative with your words, as author Peter McWilliams wrote in, "*You Can't Afford the Luxury of a Negative Thought.*"[6]

Speak empowering value and virtue based words. This can be key to positive behavior modification, teaching and leadership. For instance, listen to the difference between these two statements: "You did a good job today" versus "I appreciate your organization skills. It made a difference with handling the added patient load today." The first statement is empty of any information. The recipient may get a boost from winning external praise, but there's no real information about how they were successful. The second statement gives value back to the recipient in the form of specific identification of what contributed to being successful.

Using value and virtue based language builds character and relationships. It is a far more accurate way to communicate then mere good-bad statements.

Coherence is a healing state that arises from synchronicity of the heart, emotions, brain, nervous system and body which improves release of DHEA and endorphins. Can you see how coherence can arise from knowing your values and synchronizing your actions, choices and communications with them? In the instant of making a positive choice, your body chemistry will *shift* into a healthy physiology and, over time, will build resilience through reinforcement. When you *shift*, you free up the energy consumed by energy-draining stress reactions and counterproductive thoughts. Then you have more energy available for the creation of health and what you desire.

Cultivation is what it takes to grow a plant. The soil, water and weather all need to be in a range that supports its healthy growth and flowering. The nutritious and fertile soil for your growth is a mix of organics from experience and lessons with value-based dreams and intentions. Speak what you want into being through empowering, value-based communication and positive action. This may seem like a lot to do, but it is more about *being*. As you weed out the thoughts that do not serve you, each moment becomes an opportunity to *choose* and cultivate a healthy way of living.

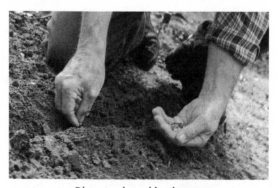

Photo in the public domain

The present moment is the perfect place and time to start. Any time you feel you miss the mark, just aim again. This cultivation of your values will build your inner resources and capacity. You become more tolerant, less likely to be host to a virus or a bad attitude that's going around your unit. You will need to affect change within and around you, project a different vibe, make different choices and attract different opportunities.

Create Nurse Influence by Choice and Decision

Are you aware, that as a nurse many eyes are on you? Yes, your patients watch every move you make, and they have long chosen you as the number-one trusted professional.[7] Your manager monitors your productivity. Since prior to 2020, the health care system has been looking to you for information and even guidance. In the last decade, metaphoric tectonic plates in the medical care model began *shifting* in the wake of decisions made in legislation about nurses and health care. You can further influence these changes and health through education, self care and wisdom, and career choices.[8]

Alan Cohen, an inspirational author and businessman, teaches that, "Every choice before you represents the universe inviting you to remember who you are and what you want."[9] This is a time to lean into your health and purpose. In the job-scape for nurses who are moving forward, each needs to do a self-inquiry and choose how they can make the most meaningful impact for health. Should the impact be in value-based purchasing or value-based living? We need nurses to influence both models, and it is timely that nurses are being asked to step up and share what they know and want, and to lead, manage and innovate.

The concepts of Yin and Yang, connection, inner wisdom, and values along with the skills of awareness, breathing and centering are foundational to building the empowerment. They will be needed for you to influence the future of nursing and health care, and your stress and health, and that of those in your care. Are you ready to act, speak and influence? Go within to change the world without. Get clear, mindfully and choose.

A message of complaint and black-lash to your employer for the hostile environment in your current workplace will probably fall on deaf ears. It will possibly close off communication and be counterproductive to this fledgling idea of listening to nurses, who are overwhelmingly women and stressed. To prepare further for this opportunity, review and relate to your past successes and potentials. The more *in-sight* you gain, the deeper your understanding, the clearer your vision, the more coherent your presence, and the stronger your voice "when speaking your mind or making a choice."[10]

Integration

With the resonance you found in your center, you may have more clarity around answers and options. Sometimes you resonate with an obvious blessing and sometimes with an unforeseen challenge that will bring a valuable lesson. Even if your choice turns out to be a more difficult path, it will have purpose uniquely for you. So ground and center, then wisely choose or re-evaluate and choose again. You have the free will to do both, at will. In this way, there are no mistakes, only opportunities, lessons and gifts.

On a new page in your journal, write "C - Choose" as the title at the top. Prepare yourself for this experience by doing the A-B-Cs.

With deepest compassion for yourself and without regrets or blame, review the positive, resonant choices revealed from your inner wisdom and center in the prior two chapters. Do any stand out in clear resonance? What does your heart choose? If you feel unable to choose, what is the reason? Repeat the A-B-Cs or at least the breathing to stay centered. Is your logical brain, rationale or reasoning interfering? Breathe and relax beyond that to your center.

You may be drawn to an option that doesn't seem to lead directly to your desired result. Intuit the balance between the associated feelings through their Yin-Yang type relationships rather than an 'either-or' method of decision-making. However, if you have specific decisions to make before choosing, such as *turn the stove off before the pot boils over*, then do so. In your mind review the previous steps in The Process for what you need: more awareness, a shift, more wisdom? It is okay to review, but try going with the guiding feeling rather than over-think.

Sometimes the choice is on a less obvious level such as continuing to work in a job that pays well, has good benefits, but exhausts you and leaves you feeling unacknowledged or unwell. The choice you have to make may not be about the job, but rather your health, yet may still lead to a different job.

Write about your options, feelings, and what of them you choose in your journal. If you perceive any difficulties, *shift* them into possibilities.

As you *shift* challenges into successes, you may be teased by fears, logistics, reasonings, and paradigms into un-serving feelings that want to keep you stuck. You still may not know what to choose, or despite having chosen, you may need to chose again. You change the world by how you choose to live in it. This is the way. The next step is to elevate. Doing so will not only help you chose, but also transform road blocks into a building blocks and stepping stones.

CHAPTER 12

ELEVATE

To elevate means to rise or lift. This important step is where you emerge from the weightiness of all the information you've been processing, and the gravity of the status quo keeping you in the stress, holding you back, trapping you in fear and doubt, or otherwise stifling your health, creativity and joy.

A change in perspective can assist with change. A higher vantage point – whether intellectual, physical, emotional or vibrational – often makes the difference in solving a problem or achieving a dream. How high is necessary? The simplest answer is 'any bit *higher* than that which created the problem' will be helpful. The concept of elevating is not limited to the linear concept of height. Instead, it is multi-dimensional and omnidirectional. Consider looking forward, backward, to either side, inside, outside, above, below and at the intersections of each. Being open, holding space and shifting are all means of changing one's perspective. It's called elevating because awareness usually follows higher conscious intentions and guidance because it reaches into possibility. In this chapter we will explore concepts and means of elevating.

Elevation fundamentally requires your willingness, intention and diligence. The biggest effort is in getting started. Like the g-force experienced with rapid acceleration, you will feel the weight of inertia, expectations, obligations, patterns and limitations increase as you build the kinetic energy for transformation. As you elevate your intention and consciousness, your vibe changes. All of your ongoing efforts synchronize becoming more efficient. Even though there is a sense of ease, at higher velocities of energy you must remain impeccable with your thoughts and words. Just as tiny movements of steering translate into big changes in direction of a car at at high speed, fleeting thoughts can quickly modify your trajectory.

Use your skills from the A-B-Cs to continue to hone your awareness, mindfulness and intention. Awareness and presence are elevations in consciousness. Integrate elevated lifestyle activities to build health such as the seven healthy habits in the diagram below.

7 Healthy Habits You Can LIVE With!

Conscious Activity: Develop an exercise routine of 20 - 30 minutes, at least three times a week. Be Present during all activity you are engaged in. Participate in activities which support life, balance and health.

Conscious Breathing: Correct breathing can clear your mind, energize your body, and make it easier to handle the unexpected or undesired.

Conscious Choices: Take an active part in your life. Realize your options. Express your self-care in the choices you make.

Conscious Eating: For your benefit and the benefit of our planet. Eat for the sake of nutrition. Replenish the earth by composting.

Conscious Gratitude: Give Thanks to your family and friends, your guides and gurus, Nature, your Higher Power, and your "Self" daily and throughout the day.

Conscious Listening: The whispers of our "being' are where the truths to our happiness and Life Purpose lay. Be still and silent for 5-15 minutes, three times each day.

Conscious Respite: Meditation or a meditative milieu will promote relaxation, clear thought, creative spontaneity and increased productivity during you activities.

©1998 Barbara Young

Breathing is the simplest way to incite elevation. Literally and metaphorically, inspiration inflates and inspires – *in-spirit-ation*. Balanced by the calming and grounding of expiration, the two phases of breathing create a vacillating polarity, a counter-balancing strength of relationship, as in Yin-Yang. Doing so will give you clarity, creativity, momentum and leverage to elevate over your stress, challenges and disappointments.

The quality of breath has a big influence on and interplays with the homeostasis of the body's electro-chemistry to raise energy and consciousness. It facilitates inner vision, clarity and wisdom. The deepest diaphragmatic and abdominal breathing actually synchronizes movements of the structural components of the body: sacrum, pelvis, spine and skull bones. The expansion, contraction, compression, rocking and oscillatory movements promotes circulation of fluids in the body. Much like the flow of energy in an electric circuit, the physics of this relates to energy flow in the form of ionic charges and discharges from the velocity and movement of electrolytes in lymph, blood and the cerebrospinal fluid (CSF). Intentional breathing techniques, such as those done in various yoga poses and practices, can contribute to the body's flow of energy and build the electromagnetic field. This field has aliveness and is interactive. You may sense this within yourself and around others as low energy, magnetic personality, a glow or hyper energy.

Do the A-B-C technique now while seated or lying down. Use deep, prolonged, diaphragmatic breathing on exhalation and inhalation. Deepen your awareness and explore the movement of the air into the recesses of your sides and back, throat and sinuses. Feel your breath move up and down your spine like a rolling wave following your spinal curves, massaging abdominal organs and enhancing lymphatic flow. Feel the multidimensional expansion and contraction of the abdomen and chest, the curl and uncurling of tailbone and cervical-spine, the elongation and recoil of the spine, and the sense of expansion, lightness and settling within your awareness. You may discover a rocking movement within your body and posture that feels comforting.

Observe and breathe – relaxed, slow and deliberate. Inhalation and exhalation are prolonged for this activity.

Squeeze the lower abdominal muscles at the end of expiration to completely empty. This can mimic the response from a Valsalva maneuver generating gentle back-pressure that refers upward through your throat, soft palate and head, and stimulates a special endocrine gland in the center of the brain, called the pineal gland. It is important for circadian rhythm regulation via the production of melatonin. It is also known as the *seat of spirit*, connecting your awareness to expansive consciousness. This helps with elevating, looking deeper into issues, and wider for new ideas, options, understanding and solutions. Breathe this way for a minute or so.

With long periods of diaphragmatic breathing, emotions can surface. This is not the purpose in this activity, however should they arise, allow them and continue to breathe. As *energy-in-motion* (emotion), they will express then empty, resulting in relief from holding onto them. In this case, take care that you are not light-headed, drink water to refresh yourself and become alert.

What do you feel during and after breathing this way? How is that different for you? How is your alertness? Level of awareness? Clarity? Energy? Describe your new state of awareness, openness or aliveness. Make brief notes about your experience of this elevated state and anything that came up for you as potential ways to resolve, release, heal and succeed.

Elevate by Breaking Habits

Think about your morning and daily routines. If you are like most, nearly the same set of thoughts and behaviors get you through any day. Many of the decisions are the same. Often activities are done in the same order and you expect your day at work to go essentially the same as usual. Your routine thoughts are not necessarily bad, some are likely necessary to cope or aid in efficiency. The effects are cumulative and stressful when caught in mundane or robotic patterns that do not lead you emotionally or professionally in a direction that you desire. To reduce this stress and resistance, infuse your life with variety and allow for spontaneity.

Try changing a few things up to break your routine:

> » Use your non-dominate hand to brush your teeth, open a door knob, or for expression as you talk.
> » Drive a different route to work and notice your experience.
> » Set an intention each morning such as choosing to be optimistic despite whatever happens that day.
> » Think of an optimistic word or phrase and use it throughout the day.

Record the variations in your journal and write about your experience before going to bed that evening. Consider how your day was different from usual. How did your intention influence the day? Did you recall your intention through the day or forget about it?

Most of your patterns and habits have become automatic or subconscious replays. These run even when you are not paying attention. Unless you intervene, they are actively creating your life as you unknowingly consent. When you become aware of a habit, stop for a moment and contemplate whether it supports your well-being or sabotages your dream.

It is possible to think, speak or act differently by choice. When you consistently interrupt the pattern and insert a new desired behavior or thought, you are *re-hab-ilitating* your *habits* by helping the brain make new neural connections. This adaptability of the brain is neuroplasticity and it builds the structural support for new habits, thoughts, and outcomes.

Elevate by Creating Your Thoughts

The *busy-ness* of routines, expectations and agendas lure you to be, do and have more, often to meet the expectations of others. At this point in the AH SUCCESS Process, you have become aware of these automatic thoughts, beliefs and habits. In terms of creativity, there is a cause and effect relationship between your consciousness and your life whether your thoughts control you or you control your thoughts.

Dr. Rick Hanson, a neuroscientist and author says, "Your brain is like Velcro for negative experiences, but Teflon for positive ones."[1] To become empowered, Dr. Hanson advises, a single breath can positively change your mental state, resulting in new neural connections, and by doing so, you own your mental state and the outcomes in your life. In this way, you are moving toward living an empowered life, the effect of your elevated thoughts, beliefs and philosophies. You elevate them by acting through the power of your choice, from your values, while aiming higher using your virtues.

Accessing your inner wisdom is an evocation of that which is within to expand your view, see a different perspective, elevate your thoughts, and potential outcomes. This *shift* from stress toward a more optimistic state *is a change* in your energy. It is upon this *shift* that you begin to resonate with the possibilities you create within.

Elevate Perspective

You may have previously heard this wisdom, "Don't judge a person until you have walked a mile in their shoes." From someone else's shoes, another perspective, things should look very different. Whether looking at your life, a situation, conflict or your career, viewing the matter from above the scene will show you a bigger picture. The practice you learned from the earlier chapters of awareness and observation of your inner self will help you elevate. Think of awareness as a narrow flashlight beam shining on the details of something right before you. Your understanding is limited in that you cannot see the whole picture. You can gain the leverage of perspective by elevating, resulting in a wider field of illumination, which changes your experience by way of possibility and *shifting* your awareness to a new perspective. Through observation, your mind's perception will have changed, as will the apparent reality of the situation because perception *is* reality. From there, you may glean new insights and achieve a new understanding, which can seem like a *re-veal-ation (revelation)*.

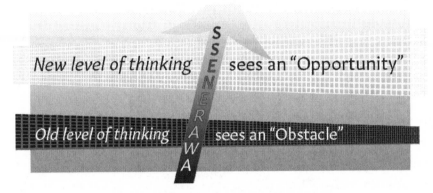

Levels of Thinking. Graphic by Vivo Digital Arts

Many astronauts have shared their surreal and elevated experience while in orbit, during their first glimpse of Earth from space. Their experience has been named, "the overview effect."[2] The astronauts describe their experience as awe.[3]

It is fairly common to hear the word 'awesome' used in everyday experiences. Though derived from the word awe, it is a pale comparison. Awesome contains 'some awe' but usually people are already on to the next thought, topic or experience mere seconds later. True awe stops you, your thoughts, your breath and your awareness of the moment. There is a reordering of relation as you likely feel smaller. This is not low self-esteem, but respectfully taking your place, merging with the whole – which is greater than the sum of its individual parts. This is not to minimize the individual because without you, the whole cannot be complete. Your separate-self fades into expansive oneness. This may sound grand, but when you elevate your perspective you, in effect, bring some awe to the situation.

The phenomenon of transcendence[4] has been intensively researched by neuroscientist Dr. Andrew Newberg since the 1990s using brain scans. He is currently Director of Research at the Myrna Brind Center for Integrative Medicine at Thomas Jefferson University Hospital and Medical College. In his recent book, *How Enlightenment Changes Your Brain: The New Science of Transformation,* written with research collaborator Mark Robert Waldman, he reveals changes in emotional and physical health that are connected to changes in the brains of people who meditate and have experienced transcendence. He highlights that a significant difference between these related states is the duration of effect and that true transcendence truly changes a person – the fabric of their being.[5] An elevated perspective helps with understanding. Meditation as a personal practice will help to elevate your perspective.

Elevate Communication

Your communication becomes less muddled by emotional overtones, when you are honest with yourself and see things from a higher perspective. You no longer unnecessarily take things so personally but rather maintain *respons-ability*. You accept your part in the matter, let others have theirs, and do what you need to do. You move away from the wounds caused by the chemistry of stress and self-defeating thoughts. Your communication is clearer and closer to the truth of the matter because integrity. Honesty and *account-ability* are part of who you are. Information will come to you that may lead to options and solutions for issues you previously could not find the voice to express, even to your manager. This comes from a unity of heart and thought, and it starts by elevating one moment, situation, opportunity or choice at a time. As you develop heart and whole body integrity, your communication becomes more coherent, your relationships, work and life more unified and whole.

Elevate Care

It is a scientific fact that self-care improves overall well-being. Both exercise and massage can increase serotonin levels in your body.[6] Specifically, serotonin is increased nearly 30 percent by a massage along which also decreases stress hormones while increasing dopamine and oxytocin levels.[7] Serotonin is a confidence building hormone. Dopamine facilitates pleasure and motivates one toward achieving a reward. Oxytocin is another happy hormone, also called the 'bonding hormone'. When your happy hormones and neurotransmitters are in balance, you will be more productive, happier, experience less pain and will want to be around other people. Positive self-reflection, gratitude, visualization practices, laughter, and spending time in sunlight are other means of self-care that will enhance the healing chemistry in your mind and body, which you deserve to enjoy.

The care you give to yourself will affect all that you do and the care you provide for others. Your self-care is becoming of particular interest to employers as a way to save money on medical insurance, sick days and to improve staff retention. Encouraging human resources (employees) to take care of themselves is the latest drum beat. But do employers realize that the work environment also needs to change to support your health? When you bring your elevated consciousness of self-care to a supportive work environment, you will be better prepared to meet the demands with resilience and potentially have a more positive influence on patient care outcomes.

Think about your last day or work shift when you felt tired, too busy and like you needed time away from you job, but pushed through anyway. How did it go? Imagine how it would have been different for you if you had been honest and asked for help or called in sick for the day off? What if you then had a massage, a nutritious meal or a long, soothing bath instead? I know this doesn't sound realistic, but what *if* you did one of these things? Imagine how it would help or make a difference for you? If you can imagine it, you are on your way to making it happen. Make notes in your journal in response to these questions. Also note any other things that add challenges to your day, such as the amount of sleep you get, along with ideas of what you can do for self-care.

Elevate at Work

If your workplace is common, it is by its nature a venue for higher conscious learning. This is because it's a challenging environment which necessitates growth. Elevating during your work day will reduce your fatigue and experience of stress because you can put space between you and the stress. This in no way condones a better-than-thou attitude. Rather, equanimity, because you seek unity, not division through improved communication and team work. It will help you be more organized, efficient and enhance cognitive function. It's challenging to raise your head up from the trenches and see the space to do anything beyond what your assignment requires, but do take the time to do so. Look out the window at the blue sky or leaves dancing in the wind. Connect with a colleague through a smile, nod or perhaps with a pat on the back to boost moral and team cohesiveness.

You will get better at this the more you practice the skill. Even practicing in home situations will help you be more skillful doing it at work. Some things happen in the moment, such as a physiological *shift* from intentional breathing or by taking a break, and some things build over time, such as resilience and your ability to see new options.

You work in the physical world, but the energetic world dwells in you and effects the physical world. Conscious awareness of this is elevating. Here are a few ways to facilitate elevating during a stressful work day or when there is work overload, conflict or disagreeable interactions:

- Be the observer – step back from a situation
- Ask an option-provoking question
- Pause to allow space
- Breathe
- Swallow to relax your throat, jaw and tongue
- Drink water
- Change your physical position
- Take a break
- Meditate
- Go for a brisk walk
- Step out for fresh air
- Connect with the a caring feeling in your heart.

The resistance to break away from the rhythm and pace of work or pull yourself out of a power struggle can be immense, and studies show you will be sharper after you do. Simply become aware, breathe and center. It may help to say to yourself, "stop" or "unplug" to command your attention, while quickly imagining the *plug* of your nervous system being removed from the *socket* of the situation. You can then plug into your inner wisdom, which will help you elevate to sense the real or bigger issue.

By changing the level of your thinking, the dynamics of your interactions will be influenced. Having *shifted* within, you can influence the milieu in your unit.

Elevate Environment

Has your work organization presented concepts for promoting a positive work environment, a culture of safety or patient-centered care? There is likely a list of values somewhere in their literature as well. Become familiar with them if you did not already do so in Chapter 10. Look for the ones that are shared and any connections between their values and your virtues identified in the same chapter. Express these in your job and use the words to show merit or remedy in a work situation.

Acknowledge innovation, reward compassion and tell a colleague you admire their integrity. Active integration of your employers' values and your virtues into work flows, care delivery and *inter-hierarchical* communication is a way which these concepts can come into *real-ization*.

You are already a leader in this culture, even as you think you have no power or influence. Elevate your thinking to see your place as a member of the number-one trusted professionals, voted for nearly two decades by people in the community who trust nurses to maintain their best interest as the priority.[8] Your employer is fortunate to have you working with them.

(💮) Did you feel a *shift* inside or an elevation in perspective when you read that you are the "number-one trusted professional"? Pause here and breathe while you experience that. It is beyond a verbal compliment or statistic, it is an affirmation. Recognize this within yourself. Feel affirmed and gracious.

What does it feel like to receive this merit? What comes up for you when experiencing this acknowledgement? What within you feels challenged by the thought of being influential, including anything making it difficult to receive any ideas or inspirations for modulating your work environment?

For a nurse, any breech, in their sacred relationship and unspoken honorable agreement with patients causes moral injury. How can nurses recover and protect this vital yet disregarded pillar of nursing care as irreplaceable *technology* where time or cost driven methodologies dominate? Write about these things in your journal.

Elevate the Paradigm

Even with a well-defined framework of principles and practices, beliefs and lore to make up a paradigm, there is inherently space or potential. As in the universe itself, the tangible amounts to far less than the space contained within it. Gloria Steinen said, "God may be in the details, but the goddess is in the questions. Once we begin to ask them, there's no turning back." Because a tightly woven paradigm leaves little space for possibility, growth or expansion, it can become inflexible and limited like a box.

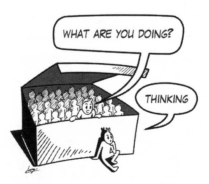

Graphic by the author, art by Lang

Let's explore this from a higher level while keeping in mind the symbol and concept of Yin and Yang. As the seed of Yin is within the fullness of Yang, mainstream nursing care is imbedded into the medical model of care with its highly specialized diagnostic algorithms and specialized interventions. These are aimed at treating symptoms, disease and trauma largely at the tangible, structural and chemical levels. This expert yang model-based system implicates separateness through specialization, while functionally minimizes holistic understanding. Holism is not about singularity, it is about wholeness through relationship and diversity.

Unfortunately, simply including the patient in the center of the model, as the one who receives attention from multiple disciplines of practice, may look like it's wholistic in a drawing, but it is deficient in the integration of and balance from other dimensions of understanding. Patients have frequently verbalized to me their frustrations and feelings of insignificance within this model. Further, they expressed feeling their care was fragmented, as if they had no voice and that one practitioner didn't speak to another. Perhaps the "nurse navigator" roles that appeared in the mid twenty-teens, for guiding patients through their treatment, are a step in a balancing direction. If their job descriptions give them the leeway, the nurse navigators can aid in personalizing care, raising the voice of the patients, and facilitating continuity of care through improved communication. Particularly if the nurses who are in the navigator roles learn, model and teach the principles of holism, epigenetics and self-regulation.

As the modern scientific perspective advances, it expands the bounds of the known into what was previously unacknowledged, yet existed. Science has revealed new, more inter-related patterns that confirm connectedness, universality, unity, and oneness, including on the level of the unseen. An elevation in thinking for the modern medical model might highlight relationships and interactions between everything, including nutrition, events, body organs, systems, toxins, health and environments.

Healthcare is burdened by the effects of the societal separation from health promoting lifestyle and social services that facilitate health.

"The United States does not have a health care system," according to Rebecca Onie, chief executive of the Boston-based group Health Leads, instead it has a "sick care system".[9] This may be shocking to hear said so clearly, but she backs her point by the fact that vastly more resources are apportioned to after-illness treatments. What would the spectrum of health and illness look like if we took her challenge to truly take care of health?[10] This in no way discounts the need for expert care of illness and early disease screening, but health needs to be tended to and facilitated as *the* goal.

Elevate Health

An elevated perspective of health reveals it is more than the assessment of acceptable physical metrics and care involves more than treating symptoms as they occur. Experiencing symptoms and stress seems normal in the modern way of life because it is normal for the body to produce messages of distress (symptoms) when suffering from neglect or being threatened (fight or flight). But that 'normal' is not natural because what is natural is to be healthy and resilient. Health is a multi-dimensional state of being unified and wholesome that people in modern-day life can and must cultivate.

The healthcare paradigm must shift to embrace a more proactive perspective of caring for health as a way of life from birth. When health is elevated, there is increased likelihood for more health to be created, in people, the environment and economics.

Elevate Nurse Leadership

Looking deeper into what is needed to elevate the current paradigm, it is necessary to elevate people. People need information, a voice, a choice, access and influence over their lives, health and health care, all of which nurses can provide or facilitate. Nurses and the people working in the healthcare hold the power to accept the challenge of choosing change or to continue paying for an outdated paradigm with their health. Individually and collectively they can *shift* their perspectives from brain to heart, stress to success, and illness to health.

Nurses traditionally are agents of positive change and can lead this *shift* from internal empowerment instead of the voice of their inner frustrated nurse who usually attends the staff meetings. Ralph Waldo Emerson said, "Treat a man as he is, and he will remain as he is. Treat a man as he could be, and he will become what he should be." This is what you as a nurse do in your relationship with people and patients. Together, you transcend limitation and circumstance. This is why I say you are "the conduit of care." No matter how technical the procedure you are doing, first and foremost you are the conduit or connection to the person behind patient-label and to their heart. You are there to treat your patients in light of their full potential (elevate) and not as a diagnosis, treatment, procedure, statistic or billing code.

As a healthy, self-empowered, creative, influential nurse, your care elevates the current medically-based paradigm, you provide the balancing yin perspective not attainable through procedures, medications or technology via the care you give. Elevating your nursing knowledge of people, relationship, human response, well-being, health and care, elevates the very things that have been lacking viability in and are being drained from the current healthcare paradigm.

What would it be like if nurse leadership and wisdom was elevated? Nurses could lead healthcare's reset. How could healthcare benefit from a metaphorical deep breath, centering with an elevation of thought, a restatement of its mission, vision and purpose, then a re-alignment of its future course toward creating health? These are beautiful questions like Warren Berger presents in *The Book of Beautiful Questions* where he asks the reader to decide, create, connect and lead. He says asking beautiful questions helps us be more engaged, fulfilled and successful leaders because they open possibilities, reveal game-changing ideas.[11] Nurses who ask beautiful questions are like Gloria Steinen's goddess, mentioned above, leading the way for the answers to be discovered.

What beautiful questions do nurses need to ask? How can nurses inspire healthy people and influence caring for health? How do you see this done currently or why isn't it done? What if you could create health for yourself, inspire healthy people and influence caring for health? How would that look? How would each day feel if you created health all day? What is a healthy lifestyle? What is a healthy environment? Describe any inter-relatedness you realize between health, lifestyle and environment. These are important questions to contemplate. What would the health-care system and paradigm look with a healthy balance of nursing wisdom, caring for health? How does changing the word healthcare into two words – health care – change the meaning? Write freely about your answers, ideas and questions in your journal.

Elevate Energy

The research results of modern science are advancing paradigms in major influential *shifts* that, if allowed, will elevate energy as a predominant factor in health and healing. Not only in medical interventions, technological innovations and computing, but in the concepts of *shifting* consciousness and energetics of healing. Remarkable heart-based scientific advancements are giving reason for our conscious minds to embrace intuition, energy and electromagnetics in our self-care, well-being and paradigm. The merger of the predominant Western health-care paradigm and those of ancient wisdoms may not be possible, but that doesn't negate either one. It is possible for a harmonious holistic paradigm, to evolve where each has purpose as in the principal of Yin and Yang. To achieve this, health as the intention, must be strengthened through active expression in life. These yin aspects lie with people, and nurses.

Energy flowing in a biological system is necessary for life. In the body, energy is created for physical activity, emotions and cellular processes of biology via chemical, mechanical, electrical, magnetic and photosynthetic means.

An electrical charge is a quality related to the flow of energy via the movement of electrons or ions that results in impulses of energy. You may recall the electrical charge is created by the sodium-potassium pump across cell membranes. Our nervous system depends upon the distribution of such ions to create electrical impulses. Cardiac cells generate the energy for contraction and the heart generates an electromagnetic field. You have likely seen sparks of light when you've bumped your head or by merely squeezing your eye lids closed as the pressure on the nerves releases flares of light (energy). Our bodies also build up, carry and discharge static energy from friction and stress. High energy emotions have the charge and voltage to attract, excite and fight.

The body also responds to electricity and electromagnetic frequencies (EMFs). Electrical stimulation to muscles can override pain signals in the nervous system or cause tetany in the muscle. Bone tissue is piezoelectric, which means it stores electrical energy that is released when mechanical pressure is applied. Because of this amazing natural ability, researchers are discovering that precise electrical stimulation shows promise in helping bones heal.[12] Further, electromagnetic frequencies in the environment can change hormone-release in the brain and cause nerve excitation affecting mood and energy levels. And, there are little factories in each cell called mitochondria, that convert energy from nutrition, water and light into energy for the body. Depletion of energy at this level can lead to cell death, likened to the manifestations occurring in the critical stage of exhaustion of Hans Selye's General Adaptation Syndrome.[13]

Amazingly, each of the trillions of cells in your body has the ability to create, store, transmit and receive energy.

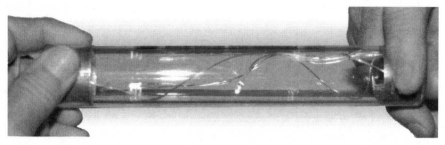

Lights shine, powered by the energy circuit created when two people hold an end of tube in one hand and then touch each other with the other hand.
Photo by Barbara Young

In the integrative healing arts classes I co-taught at a community hospital in Northern California, I presented information about energy. Nurses received it with a range of acceptance from respectful curiosity to curiously skeptical. I imagine that you may be in that range too. To help demonstrate, I used a working model of a circuit in a closed ended, clear plastic tube with lights, wires and a battery contained inside. It operated without an on-off switch. I asked the group to hold hands and form a circle. Randomly, I asked two people to let go of their joined hands. One held one end of the tube. Then the other completed the circle again by holding the other end of the tube. At the moment the circle was complete, so was the circuit. The participants gasp at what happened – lights flashed and there were musical sounds. The group usually tried to trick the gadget by breaking contact or touching each other with varying degrees of pressure which caused the lights to go off, dim and brighten along with the crescendo and decrescendo of music. The model circuit was responsive because the human body conducts electricity.

Are you willing to *shift* and elevate to discover even more of your personal power through discovering and managing your energy?

⊗ Breathe in and exhale to relax and become aware. Hold your hands in front of you with flat palms facing at 1-2 inches apart. Play with the distance. Do you sense anything between your hands...temperature, movement, density, sensations? This is radiant or thermal energy from your body. Move them in smooth rotations around their position, maintaining the palms facing and apart. Do this for a minute. You might start to feel sensations in your palms. It may feel warm and tingling, and involve your fingertips as well. You may feel a thickness or cushion develop.

You can play with this sensation, moving palms back and forth, toward and away from each other. How far apart can you separate your hands and still experience the sensations? Roll the sensation between your palms like you would to round snow into a ball. This rotating motion stirs the activity of the electrons. To intensify the sensations, rub your palms together briskly about a dozen times. Then stop with palms still facing and separate your palms slightly. What happens? How does it feel? Bring your palms toward each cheek and hold them about a half-inch away. Feel the sensation on your cheeks.

Write in your journal about your observations and experiences of your body's energy during these exercises.

Elevate Electromagnetics

A field refers to an area under the influence of a force, such as that which comes from a magnet, your heart or intention. You have a field of energy surrounding your body that communicates with *The Field* of energy and information which contains and connects all things, including the field of your loved ones and the Earth.[14] This may be a challenge to wrap a traditionally-educated brain around if one is not familiar with this information.

Attempt to elevate to this possibility and consider what would affect change at the level of these fields? Emotions, intentions, electric and magnetic influences? Science has proven that our bodies contain electromagnetic generators, of which the heart is the most powerful. Here in lies inner *technology*, more profound than the emerging man-made 'internet of things', capable of affecting change at both local and remote distances.[15] Intentions are influential. Breathe and increase your capacity of space held for the possibility that states of your brain and heart do affect life on the level of *The Field*.

(♡) Let's work with the energy of your heart's electromagnetic field. First, use one hand, palm flat. Bend your arm at your elbow, bringing a flat palm toward your face, and touch your lips with flat fingers. Pause, then straighten your elbow, which will move your fingers away from your mouth and outward. What was that like? Did you experience anything? There were muscular contractions and relaxation, flexion, extension and rotation. Did you get it? If not, it's okay. Do it again, but first, *shift* your awareness, via your breath, to the area around your heart in the center of your chest. As you breathe, increase your awareness of any sense of warmth in this area and any emanations from your heart.[16]

Next, think of someone you care about and picture them a distance away, maybe getting in the car to go to work for the day. Feel a heart-based emotion or virtue such as compassion, care, friendship or love in the area in your chest. Continue to feel that feeling as you smile and think about your person. Do you feel the energy shifting within you and from you? The warmth moves upward into your face as you smile, it glows outward and extends toward your someone. The palm of your hand may tingle as you bestow an energetic blessing upon them and wave to them. Maybe you are compelled to touch fingers to your lips and transfer the radiating heart energy that is flushing your face and warming your lips such that it sparks onto your fingers, so hot you quickly hurl it to them. Wow! Feel that? Feel your outstretched hand and arm amplify your heart's radiance outward to reach them.

Be here for a few minutes. Feel the connectedness of this. What just happened? Notice how you feel. This is an example of an electrical and magnetic occurrence. Imagine how this loved one feels after receiving the energy from you. See them in your mind and feel their ease, joy, healing or other meaningful experience. Experience receiving the kiss they blow to you as they drive off. Experience how it ignites your feelings. Be aware of the interconnection and imagine how they feel carrying your presence with them throughout their day.

When ready, *shift* your breathing and awareness back to reading this book, noticing what changes for you. Feel any variations of intensity, temperature, levity, anything you can notice. Make notes in your journal about your experience. Do you still feel that heart-based emotion as you write? What are your thoughts about what you just did?

You have just sent energy to your loved one. In the above Heart Activity, you intentionally transmitted vibrations of thoughts and energy from the magnetic field that emanates from your heart and envelopes your body into a realm that is also accessible by your special someone. This exemplifies the quantum perspectives involving *The Field* and entanglement, the connectedness of all things. This progressive science has discovered answers to many of your questions, but no doubt you can feel this is a major shift in perspective from the usual everyday perceived reality.

How does your energy and information travel in *The Field*? Take a breath as you open to possibilities. There is no separation of space and time; they are concurrent in the quantum world between you and your person. In this realm, *now* is the only moment. Nowhere becomes 'now here.' There is no distance to travel, because quantum physics holds, that all things are unified in *The Field*, not only connected, but also entangled. This means what happens to one, happens to the other and the whole. This is why you can feel the pain of another. Further, everything is *no thing*. Rather, in *The Field* from which everything arises, all is expressed as energy and information, traveling into our perceived reality in waves of light, sound, frequency and thought. You have special neurons in your brain called mirror neurons that sense this information and cause the experience within you. These enable you to imitate, learn and empathize.[17] Though not all of this energy and information is sustained into a dense, tangible manifestation, it is no less real. Modern physics has proven that the character of physical reality is largely beyond the range of visible experience. Just like the full light spectrum of which only a very narrow section is visible to the human eye. There is a non-local reality that underlies the perceived solid reality of form and structure.[18] This is the connectedness of all things that are seen as separate. "*The Field*," as Einstein concisely stated, "is the only reality."[19]

When you looked for your awareness in Chapter 6, did you ever find it? Yet you experience it and know of it within your body and being. With focus, you can localize your awareness but cannot find it located anywhere tangibly. Similarly, quantum physics describes that energy appears to have form when observed (localized) and it is this perspective from observing that makes it appear solid. The moment attention is directed away, it becomes a formless. So when you focus your attention, your awareness becomes clear to you, because it presents what you think about. This perception is your *real-ity*. When you align your thoughts, feelings and emotions, especially within the range of heart-felt emotions, not only is the frontal lobe of your brain enhanced, you *shift* into coherence. You are generating an electromagnetic influence which emanates into and positively affects your external environment via *The Field* which constitutes *real-ity*. Just as important to understand is this coherence and influence happens with negative and stressed emotions too. Just like when you wake up sleep-deprived and grumpy and every seems to go wrong, especially thing that you touch. You know how this day goes – you catch every red light on the way to work, your computer crashes, no meds arrive on time for administration and your patients seem demanding.

We cannot underestimate that which we do not yet understand. 'Existence' vacillates between the seen and unseen. Awareness and perception facilitate growth as you learn and see what you didn't previously. Remember the crack that lets the light of possibility in? There are cracks in conventional knowledge and room for further understanding in the area of energetics. Energy Medicine and the new field of research called Neurotheology are revealing deeper understanding.[20] Hold space for positive possibility and let your heart light shine.

Elevate Connection

The Global Coherence Monitoring System registers the magnetics of planet Earth around the world as part of the international effort of The Global Coherence Initiative (GCI) launched in 2008 by the Institute of HeartMath. The GCI seeks to help activate the heart of humanity and promote peace, harmony and a *shift* in global consciousness.[21] This is important because of the connectedness of all things. The Earth's magnetic fields affect and sustain life and health on Earth, which is why time spent surrounded by nature and grounding are beneficial to people. Now there is proof that our emotions and energy field affects those of our planet.

The largest electromagnetic spikes ever recorded were on September 11, 2001. These began about 15 minutes after the first plane hit the World Trade Center building in New York City and continued to increase for several hours after. The magnetometers detected the drastic changes in the earth's magnetic fields that produced seismograph-like spikes. These revealed the dramatic influence on the Earth's energy field from the intense collective emotional experience of large and growing numbers of people as the news spread around the world.

Gregg Braden, author, scientist and internationally renowned pioneer in bridging science, spirituality and human potential, summarizes that this data dispels two assumptions the dominant thought system in the West has been based upon.

- All things are separate and cannot influence each other.

- Our inner world of thought, feeling, emotion and beliefs cannot influence the outer world.[22]

The electromagnetic spikes described above are a clear demonstration of a human energetic connection, the collective influence of people, and human connection with our environment and planet – each part of a continuous field that connects all things, indivisible. Does this information elevate your paradigm of life, health, relationships and environment? The heart is both a generator and a sending unit of the electromagnetic impulses of emotions felt in the heart. Thoughts are powerful and heart-based feelings and emotions, negative or positive, are even more powerful.

Imagine what holding a feeling of peace in communities of people around the world would create. This, too, has been studied and correlates with reductions in crime, emergency calls and emergency department (ED) visits.

As a nurse, your professions' paradigm is a holistic, unified, multi-dimensional human model. You work with the *technologies* of human response, awareness, choice, perspective and coherence naturally and in your work. You embody the unifying principles of heart, presence and intuition. Please take care not to lose heart from the degrading effects of stress. You are connected with all of your patients, the conduit of care. Your knowledge of health and care are vital and elevate the paradigm of the healthcare system.

Your keen awareness can detect:

- Changes in vibration that can affect mood or cause physical symptoms such as nausea,
- Force fields such as emotions, blood sugar or hormonal changes in the body,
- Pressure and temperature on the skin, ears and sinuses.

Being able to sense your own state of being is important for differentiation of what is environmentally external or internal. Environment influences your health and stress. Learning to *shift* out of a state of illness and into healthy coherence is vital to your health and success.

Elevate Level of Consciousness

There is a map of consciousness that shows vibratory calibration of levels of consciousness from shame to enlightenment. David R. Hawkins, MD PhD, developed this logarithmic scale by using Applied and Behavioral Kinesiology (muscle) testing to determine the vibratory frequency of each level.[23] His scale is from one to one thousand. The numbers demonstrate sequence and progression. But the significance is the scale of their relationship. It is not arithmetic with an equal change in scale between numbers. Instead, each change is by the power of ten which is like the effect of adding a zero to the number, so "10" becomes "100" which becomes "1000" and so on.[24]

These numbers are describing a vibratory frequency. So to elevate your consciousness you have to *raise your emotional vibration.* Should a situation de-energize you, from this information perhaps you can gain insight into why you feel the deceleration, depression, fatigue or weakness as your vibration lowers. The level you identify with isn't meant to be a label you wear, but a way to understand your experience, emotions, challenges, stress, and gifts.

While you can *shift* between these states throughout the day, or one may dominate different situations for you in life, Dr. Hawkins claims we each have a core level of functioning. Knowing your core level helps you understand your personal growth. You likely have a sense of your character (core) and can sense when your expression is more or less than the capacity you usually display. You may generalize it to being a pessimist or optimist, but this scale provides more information. It reveals a potential for elevating your awareness, thought, and actions through resonance.

By now you are getting more comfortable going within yourself for clues and answers, using the Easy as A-B-C technique. This is where you will understand your core level of consciousness if you are open and willing to know and be honest with yourself. Then you can intentionally set out to build your capacity and elevate. Your emotions enliven or weaken your muscular, immune, central nervous, digestive, hormonal and cardiovascular systems...your overall health.

⊚ As you read about each level of consciousness described in the text below, attempt to feel it or recall an experience of it. Make notes in your journal, but particularly notice how you experience the different levels. See if you can sense the *shifts* in energy and if you recognize your core level of consciousness.

Have you ever felt shame? If so, its likely you will not have to go very deep into the experience to recall the drained feeling of powering down to this level. This is the lowest of emotional states according to Dr. Hawkins' scale, which is a costly drain on your body's resources and reserves. It cannot support health with its calibration of below 30. If you experience shame and do not process it and move through; it can be perilously toxic. If you have challenges with this issue, please consider working on this with a professional.

Fear is the primitive emotion that the stress response is based upon. It calibrates at 100. Your patients likely dip in and out of this experience frequently. Having job-related stress can bring you down to this level, but the chronic normal day of being over worked, under supported with productivity and acuity expectations and demands can also trigger the stress response and physiology of fear. This is not a healthy vibration if it is sustained or frequently episodic. Look at the scale and see how far de-energized it is from other desirable states.

The emotions associated with grieving span from fear to courage. These emotions can feel near crippling, but they are necessary to process and climb back toward living with courage again.

Courage is at 200. Dr. Hawkins equates this to the first level of empowerment because you *shift* out of fear, vulnerability and taking energy from other people and situations. This is a completely different state, beyond circumstance and external validation when you accept that you are *response-able* for your growth and achievement.

Willingness is 310. During a stressful work shift, each moment you spend feeling a state of willingness (flexibility), especially in your heart and body, you are raising your vibration into a positive state that makes a foundational contribution toward building your resilience.

Based on the levels of consciousness from David Hawkins, MD.[25]
Graphic by Vivo Digital Arts

There is a level of consciousness called reason, calibrated at 400, which Dr. Hawkins says is the level of science, medicine and the desire for knowledge. Your job demands efficient reasoning for safety and proficiency. This is a yang component that must be balanced with sensitivity for nurses to be present with their patients as the conduit of care. But functioning solely or predominantly by reason can draw you down from the levity of higher emotions.

Love is the next level at 500, just below the level of sainthood, on the way to enlightenment. You enter into the vibration of love only when you rise above reason in service to the good of mankind, letting the heart take over rather than the mind, and live by intuition. I see the deep calling of a nurse to be at least at this level, particularly in the rugged terrain of today's healthcare.

After reading and experiencing this information, you may begin to comprehend why certain thoughts and experiences cannot come to you at certain levels and why they easily occur at others. For more understanding of the Scale of Consciousness, it's important to read Dr. Hawkins' book, *Power vs. Force*. ⓘ

Elevate Your Unit

Dr. Hawkins proposes that everything in our environment can affect our level of consciousness:

- Sounds, including both volume and intensity, industrial noise, tone of voice and type of music.
- Information we deal with such as books, news, diagnoses and treatments.
- Those we associate with at work, in our family, friends and communities.

In the work environment, labeling stock and creating nurse oriented work flows, along with ergonomic evaluations of equipment, lighting, and noise level, and removing clutter are a few things that might be promptly done. Building a cohesive and coherent team of colleagues is fundamental to elevating your unit, which influences productivity, the care you give and *shifting* from stress.

As you regulate your stress response and build energy levels, cognition and health, your colleagues will benefit from your presence. When perspectives *shift* from competition to co-efficiency, there is a multiplier effect of working together. When the team elevates together, generally hostility, complaining, gossiping and skipping breaks will reduce. Moving from one level of consciousness to the next provides more momentum and influence than found in a stepped linear progression. As consciousness increases, associated vibration (energy) and mass (influence) increases and it proportionately offsets more of the lower level life-depleting things like negativity and stress. As your team lifts up, the intricacies of communication, understanding, tolerance and respect cannot help but improve. Together the team becomes a force without the need to be forceful. You have power and influence by presence and higher intention. It starts within you.

When nurses experience long term, grave stress, it is not sustainable. Healing the work environmental imbalances and personal responses to them will modulate toward less stress and more health for nurses. Ideally, create and maintain compassion and health for and within yourself first, then model those positive attributes for those in your care and in your unit. Caring for yourself may slow the rate of illness entering into a severely burdened system. *Compassion heals the giver and the receiver.*

What if nurses, as a population, would each meditate, shift from stress to success, cultivate the electromagnetics of their heart and raise their level of thinking to that of empowerment and positive influence? How would sharing these practices with co-workers benefit your unit? How could nurses then influence health and care?

If you taught your patients to shift out of stress and raise their vibration, how might that influence the course of their treatment, the outcomes, the potential for deep healing? Imagine the collective consciousness that would be cultivated with you, your colleagues and patients. (Obviously this would not be appropriate for all patients.)

Use your journal to write down and explore these possibilities.

Elevate Your Life

There is persistence and ongoing learning involved with elevating your life, starting with expression of your virtues, and often by simply letting go. If you have not resolved something from your past, it is baggage and it weights you down.

ⓥ Meditation is an easy and ancient way to find space between your thoughts or any commotion affecting your inner world. The process leads to peace of mind and resets your mindset as you go within. It is as easy as A-B-C. Do this now. "Awareness, Breath, Center" can be used as a quick reset, or as a lead in for a longer meditation. When you find yourself in a space of awareness from meditation, see a picture or create a word to describe how you feel, such as *peace, ease, or ocean.* At any time you need a boost, a reset or a quick mental getaway, recall your picture or word, and feel the experience instantly.

Meditation will help you see your challenges, circumstances, relationships, and stress differently. You can bring a question into meditation and observe new possibilities or answers. Meditation can assist you to release, relax, *shift and* connect to your intuitive inner wisdom. Spend another few minutes in meditation. Note your experience in your journal. ⓘ

In the work you do as a nurse and in life, circumstances can drain you in an instant or can relentlessly pull down upon you. Having the wisdom to recognize when you do not understand the forces at play or that their purpose is beyond your mental comprehension invites you to seek serenity.

These are instances for giving a blessing. A blessing comes from the capacity within your positive, heartfelt emotions. Blessing something acknowledges the crack and the light. It is the light within you that honors the light within the crack, even if it is not comprehensible or visible. Through each relationship, it is possible for all to be healed and made whole. Use of blessing can be elevating.

Think of something that stresses you that needs blessing: a situation, co-worker, policy or manager. Visualize it and, for a moment, experience the helplessness or frustration, the hypocrisy or disparity, the pain or regret. Unplug yourself to remove the charge or pain of the situation. Elevate to a higher perspective to view and bless the situation. Let it be and open to becoming aware of something valuable from this situation. *Listen* for your inner wisdom to reveal something that will lift and carry you beyond this situation, creating a wholeness that acknowledges the Yin and the Yang, the two sides of every situation, the challenge and the lesson. Write about how this was for you and any *re-veal-ation*.

You might create a blessing for a situation that presents frequently, which is something that I did. I created the blessing below for patients in my care who were to receive chemotherapy, but were scared, tired, overwhelmed, feeling uncertain or defeated by their ill health. It may have been their first treatment or their twenty-first. I shared this blessing with them: "Bless this medicine. Let it only do good. Bless this body. Let it use what it needs and release what it should."

What do you experience from reading my blessing? Think of a situation that needs your blessing and write one in your journal. How do you feel different by simply writing it? Now with intention, visualize and do the blessing. How do you feel? If you find it helpful, apply it in your life.

Remember, these are a few of the feelings that elevate life when generated in the heart and felt in the body:

- Appreciation
- Beauty
- Care
- Compassion
- Forgiveness
- Gratitude
- Love

As you sustain these feelings in your heart, body and being, you feed the wellspring inside of you, replenishing yourself. It is from your overflowing cup that you can sustainably give to others.

Elevate using Forgiveness and Gratitude

Forgiveness is for giving. The blessing is that you get that which you give forward – the release. When you hold someone in a negative light, it holds you with them because you are the one holding them in that space. They will not be held without you to hold them in blame or shame. You cannot escape the bind because you have made this relationship with them in this way. Once you relate differently, your relationship with them can change.

This is a great way to fall asleep, with peace and at ease. The neurochemistry of forgiveness is restful and healing. When your mind and body are at ease during sleep, the cells and systems are balancing, detoxifying and repairing more efficiently, and you awaken more refreshed.

FORGIVENESS: Every night before falling asleep find least three people, situations or ways that you can grant forgiveness. These can be forgiveness for yourself, the driver who cut you off, your car for breaking down and making you late, or the weather for not bringing much needed rain. The purpose here is to really let go into this new way of being. Release the hold of judgment, disappointment and anger. Release the feelings of powerlessness and uncertainty. Release anything and all that you possibly can.

If you can further hold space, reflect and shift your perspective to allow a lesson to present. This will facilitate a deeper forgiveness by way of acceptance of the gift from the situation.

If you find it helpful, you can involve your body in forgiveness. If you feel an associated tension or tightness in your body, then focus on easing that area as you forgive. Or you could hold your fists tightly closed and, as your

forgive, open them and imagine the object of your forgiveness floating away free and relieved of your grip. It also
may help to shake out your hands, then sigh deeply. Exhale
fully. Say "peace" as you release the hold on the person,
thing or situation to emphasize the release of energy that
was bound in the mental constriction.

Feel the tension leave and linger with the experience of
ease that will follow. You just let go. There is no need to
ever pick up it again. Open your eyes, feel your sense of
self. See your life as it is, free and full of potential. Make
notes in your journal about your experiences with forgiveness in this exercise.

Gratitude is a gracious attitude. Attitude is something you can
choose. You have likely felt the emptiness of a token, barely audible
'thanks' or 'sorry'. Gratitude is not about the words being said, but the
intention and feeling associated with them. A weak effort conveys minimal sincerity. When you give gratitude, you must cultivate the feeling
within yourself and it is given by emanating it towards the receiver. You
know the difference and have felt it. You get what you give when you
give gratitude.

GRATITUDE: Every morning, when you awaken, express
gratitude for three things. The best thing to do upon
awakening is to sustain that momentary refreshed state just
prior to any thought. It may take practice to notice this
time period. After dwelling in this brief state, choose your
first thought and make it one of gratitude or other virtue.
You can be thankful for the new day, your breath, job or
for not feeling pain in that moment. The purpose here is to
fill your cup and set a positive resonance for your day.

When you express your gratitude, feel the sensations of
gratitude in your body and being. Does the space around
your heart warm and expand? Do you feel the energy as a
flush in your face or warmth in your body? How do you

feel the energy? What is your experience from this?

Imagine who or what you are grateful for in front of you and feel the warmth and tingling of gratitude radiating outward from you to them. Are your facial muscles at ease? Are you smiling? What is the feeling around your eyes, heart and breath? Taking this deeper into healing, you could send gratitude to the person or situation you previously released with forgiveness. Why? Because in this connected universe, every relationship has purpose. You can thank them for helping you learn forgiveness. Make notes in your journal about your experiences with gratitude.

This is a great way to start the day, warmed and filled with gratitude. It will elevate your thinking and influence your day positively. If something disturbs your bliss during the day, deal with it. If you can, find the gift offered within an incident or simply recall something you are grateful for. Cultivate that feeling in your heart. You can do this in an instant. This is mindful practice of gratitude and doing so builds sustainable resilience for well-being.

You may find it is helpful to keep a journal of these miracle moments of forgiveness and gratitude. It may become a valuable keepsake and also a soulful balm to review when you need a lift in spirit.

Integration

Are you seeing how it is necessary and possible it is to elevate? Your *respons-ability* is enhanced by changing perspectives and the resulting new choices. Use the Heart Activity that follows to give you other tools regarding the concept of elevate.

On a new page in your journal, write "E - Elevate" as the title at the top. Prepare yourself for this experience by doing the A-B-Cs.

Where are you on the scale of consciousness? What do you want to elevate to? What virtues, thoughts, words and actions synchronize with your aspiration? Write them down.

How does it feel for you to be at that desired level. Experience yourself as such and look at your previously unmanageable situation (stress) from the new level. Watch it play out from an elevated observer perspective. Can you glean the outcome? What new alternatives and choices arise? Spend time considering them as they apply to your situation and make the choices that you can. Feel your successful self regulation, how a part of you answers to your choices and rises up, committing to your success.

Do feel lighter, excited or charged? Spend time with your enlightened awareness around this. Entertain the possibilities and feel grateful for being freed from what ever appeared to trap you. Linger with this, come know your feeling of your success as your vision sharpens and your *picture* comes into focus. Make notes in your journal about your *picture* and feelings of success.

If you feel depleted or need strength or guidance to help you elevate, here are a few techniques that might help you in the moment with various circumstances. Be mindful as you do these individual and progressive postures, noticing how you feel prior to and following each of these. When performed in sequence, notice the additive effect of each movement. You may choose to do any or all as one continuous flow of movement. Make notes of your insights after doing these postures.

1. Enjoy a diaphragmatic breath. This is a relaxing technique you should be well familiar with by now.
2. Ease your shoulders and relax your jaw. This is disarming and relaxing. It also can relieve fatigue.
3. Look upward with your eyes. This is an elevating posture, like looking above the situation toward higher guidance.

4. Turn your palms up as if feeling the sun's warmth radiating upon them. You may feel tingling on your palms and fingers. Receive the *soul-ar* energy from the sun into your palms, as do the green leaves of a plant.

5. Raise your arms up, extending your elbows, with palms up and hands above and to either side of your head. Your arms should be open and forming a bowl. If you are standing (grounded), this is what I call the chalice pose. Look upward, breathe and feel the sun radiating energy, filling the bowl between your arms and down into the stem (your body) of the chalice, supported by a base (your feet) firmly connected to the earth (ground). This can be powerful as a slow intentional pose as you try to hold it as along as it takes to replenish you soul. If you are seated, you can ground through the contact with your chair that connects to the ground and feel the fullness of energy you are receiving from above and support from below.

The energy shifts quickly in mind and body as you create space for inspiration and stop feeding into frustration. The chalice pose technique involves the seven steps that we have covered so far in the AH SUCCESS Process: Awareness, Hold space, Shift, Unlock internal wisdom, Center, Choose, Elevate.

From this elevated *soul-full* state, consider the stress or matter you are working through the AH SUCCESS Process. Ask opening questions by switching from knowing to wonder. Some examples: How can this situation improve? What do I need to do to make this better? What does it feel like for me to have relief from this? By seeking and asking, you become open and your body creates a higher physiology. How does it feel different from your prior confused, angry, fearful or victim physiology? Write about your experience and answers in your journal.

Your physiology changes to follow your awareness, which changes your perception, elevating it above the level that created the problem and above any blocks. The possibilities expand and you will see ways to work through the issues and transform obstacles into tools or stepping stones.

Albert Einstein said, "There comes a time when the mind takes a higher plane of knowledge but can never prove how it got there." This is because of something else he said, "The mind will take you from point A to point B. But the imagination will take you anywhere." This happens as you elevate. It is a natural law of energy that the clearer, more resonant vibration will attract synchronization of others. This is the space you want to step into with positive action to get the success, empowerment and influence you seek.

CHAPTER 13

SEE YOURSELF WITH DESIRED RESULTS

What is seeing? What is believing? Is seeing believing? Do your eyes have to be open to see? How can seeing be important to you success?

My mom married a man with no eyes. He was a disabled veteran, with glass eyes in the sockets where his own had been surgically removed because of an infection resulting from a Vietnam War injury. When we first met, I was uncomfortable calling him blind. When I tried the word sightless, I found that really was not true. He had amazing insight, foresight and hindsight. Next I tried using the phrase, "he has no vision," but that was also far from the truth.

He had been a professional drummer, even while blind, and enjoyed being on the road, so they traveled a lot. My mom was the designated driver and he the navigator. He knew his favorite routes by heart. She knew to *let him drive* and just go with the flow. He knew the mileage and told her what speed to drive so he could calculate their time of arrival. He kept track in his head and said he could see the way in his mind. This was before GPS devices, but he had the technology within his knowing.

A major *shift* for me was when I began to accept he was blind. He had no physical eyes, but I realized it did not mean he could not see. Yes, he was physically blind, but he had vision. What he could see in his mind was his reality.

When something is lacking or blocking, we can be blind because of it. For instance, the bright sun saturates the receptors in our eyes, effectively blocking them, and we become blind as a result. If we lack particular knowledge, we may be blind to an answer. We hold values, set goals and do self care at the level of our beliefs. This is why contemplative self-inquiry can be an effective tool to elevate and improve one's ability to *see* – though our eyes can see, we can still be blind without awareness and learning.

Consider this question, "What am I refusing to accept or release that, by doing so, will serve my highest state of being and greatest good?" The answer can bring awareness. That knowledge contributes to improved understanding by removing barriers to *seeing* which creates *shifts* within.

Everyone has personally held perspectives. The likeness between these realities may lead to resonance, the differences to the opposite, dissonance. Differently held realities are the opposite of resonance, called dissonance. No doubt you have experienced dissonance, perhaps as a feeling of repulsion or a clash of perspectives with another. Our personally held perspectives blind us in our mind's eye, not only to another person's perspective, but also to options for ourselves. When we are blinded by negative, obstructive or otherwise un-serving thoughts or programming, *shifting* to a new perspective is nothing short of a miracle as we must become willing and open in order to see differently. Being willing to see things another way is how to *shift* into understanding, options, and new possibilities.

By now you likely have a sense of *something* – a feeling to go on or picture in your mind – because you have been looking inward and listening to inner wisdom. You have also been meditating and visualizing for a desired scenario. Did you use your physical eyes for any of these accomplishments? Likely not. Yet you were *seeing, viewing, visualizing or otherwise perceiving,* by way of other experiences, such as listening, feeling or *imagin-ing* – making images in your mind. Your physical senses translate information from the outside environment into impulses that become your perceptions internally. This is similar to how the transducer in an arterial line changes internal pressure information into an externally visible waveform. The realm of this interface is where magic happens.

Perception is Reality

Perception occurs on much deeper levels than that of the physical senses. Any of these deeper ways of seeing will create something vivid and dependable to guide you to your desired success or dream.

Remember that your thoughts have creative influence on your reality. In the realm of infinite possibility, your thoughts are the command. In the world of cause and effect, your thoughts cause effects in your reality.

That is why you can achieve whatever your mind can perceive. Because the neurochemistry is occurring for you to perceive, even when your mind doesn't know the difference between remembering something that happened, creating it now or imagining it happening. It's all your experience. Your mind interprets it as reality. With the engagement of your senses and feelings, you are on your way to creating it. Because of the influence of repetition, new neural pathways are created in your brain to support the new perception which will influence your thoughts, choices and actions. When you talk about it, you have added another level of creative vibration. Your felt and expressed desire adds potency. When you take concrete steps towards your dream, you are *actual-izing* it through your actions. Your dream is becoming a *real-ity* for you.

You can do this. You naturally *visual-ize* and *real-ize* all the time. Unfortunately, the human brain seems to have a negative bias making it easier to think and visualize in the negative than the positive.[1] Most people are unaware that the same creative energy is at work even when the negative, limiting and sabotaging subconscious thoughts are doing the creating. You truly cannot afford the luxury of a negative thought.[2] But the good news is that you can overcome the influence of your negative subconscious thoughts by being aware of them and choosing thoughts and values that empower. You also have the power of expectation and the placebo effect.

PHASES OF REAL-IZATION

CONCEPTUALIZE
TEND TO THOUGHTS YOU WISH TO MANIFEST

VISUALIZE
CREATE A VIVID PICTURE IN YOUR MIND

IDEALIZE
ENGAGE SENSES, DESIRE, EXPERIENCE THE FEELINGS, EXPAND VISION, AND BELIEVE

MOBILIZE
TAKE POSITIVE ALIGNED ACTION

REALIZE
STEP INTO THAT REALITY

Athletes and highly successful people use visualization. One way is to watch yourself in a movie within your mind. Another is to practice the act or presentation visually and interactively in your mind. What if you have a meeting with your manager and it is causing you anxiety? Do this visualization for a winning outcome just as an athlete might.

Get comfortable and follow the A-B-Cs to get into a relaxed and meditative state. Visualize yourself with your desired result or follow this example of having an upcoming meeting with your manager. See how you greet your manager with confidence as you arrive in her office. Feel yourself grounded and centered. See her smile at you and feel yourself smile at her. It is okay to not know what assertive-but-respectful words of clarity, integrity and unity to use at this point, just feel it happen. Continue to see the interaction from the perspective that will achieve your desired result. See you both coming to an understanding and smiling. See your heads nodding in synch, notice your posture and breathing. Look into her eyes and feel the positive feelings of having a successful meeting, communication and connection. Let this desired outcome magnetically draw you to it through the upcoming meeting. Own this outcome with gratitude, then move forward in positive aligned action, feeling as if it's already so.

If you feel resistance you can go within and inquire about it. Ask yourself exploratory questions:

» Would you rather have peace or this?[3]
» Is there something you need to release or allow?
» Is there something you need before going into the meeting?

Maybe you have met with her before and it didn't go well? If that is the case, go back to that meeting while you remain tuned in to your inner world. What can you learn from that interaction? What would you do or say or think differently?

Review that scenario in your mind and see it going well. Heal it energetically by doing what you need to do. Apologize. Rephrase your words as needed. Listen with a different ear to the intent of the communication. Learn something from it. Be centered instead of insecure. Thank her.

Feel how the situation is healed. Let that feeling flow through you and ease your mind, emotions, breath, and body. Deeply breathe in the feeling of healing. See the upcoming meeting as successful while feeling the positive energy from the prior healed meeting. Infuse it and hold the intention and space for that *real-ity*, feel gracious for it. Embody the energetics of success. Bring it through you into your next meeting and see how that is different for you. Open your eyes when you are ready.

Reflect in your journal your feelings and realizations through this activity. Having followed this example, now similarly work through it using your desired result.

In the second part of the example above you created a healing for a prior less-than-optimal situation. Through the release, you recovered the energy locked up within the unsettled encounter. Energetically you and your manager were stuck in an unhealthy pattern and it would have continued unless something *shifted*. It needed to be released for energy to flow into a different outcome. In doing so, you become a person with that success, by way of your neurochemistry and physiology, and you move forward as such. The prior Heart Activity is a linear way to walk you through a process that is quantum in nature, where *shift* and *change* can happen to bring about *desired results*.

How to Improve your Seeing

- Visualization
- Exercise your imagination
- Make your language more colorful and descriptive when you speak
- Make a collage or dream board
- Apply affirmations in present moment
- Meditate
- Cultivate self-awareness and heart-felt experiences
- Connect to your inner wisdom
- Enjoy humor
- Practice gratitude

Martha Rogers', *Nursing Theory of Unitary Human Beings*, is a validating place to start if you want to look into nursing foundations for concepts in the AH SUCCESS Process. Her theory views the unitary human being as integral to the universe and presents nursing as an art and a science directed at patterning and maintaining energy fields conducive for the patient to maximize their health potential. Health is essentially determined by the interaction between the energy fields of the human and the environment. She presents the integrality of the openness for continuous free exchange of energy, resonance and frequency.[4]

Nursing interventions are not physically invasive in the way of many medical procedures often are. However, they are often penetrating and impactful, not limited to imagery, humor, touch, music, story-telling, listening, and presence. While not used to treat symptoms or illness,they may be called for by human responses like pain and anxiety, to increase the patients' tolerance, resilience and potential for healing.

See Yourself

Does the realization of yourself as a potent energy force for your patients help reignite the light of the lamp within? Does it increase your sense of worth? Can you see a guided purpose of the path for you and your career beyond making money? What you bring to nursing and your job cannot be bottled or packaged for resale. You are the conduit for the source and the force. You are, foremost, an instrument of healing yet, by job description, a medication manager and treatment technician. The aim of your nursing work is restoring balance, wholeness and promoting health, and creating environments for health to flourish, and for relief from dissonance and disease. Cultivate the skills of heart and vision because we need heart-inspired nurse visionaries to see and create a way to a healthier future. Much of the wisdom for this can come from creating your own well-being.

> Take a moment to see, experience and feel this new refreshing perspective for yourself, your work, your relationship to your stressors, patients and colleagues, as it resonates with you. Own it. Write your exciting ideas, inspirations and visions in your journal.

Integration

You are the alchemist who transforms things for the better. The vibrational influence of your elevated perspective improves your ability to *see*. With your sensory-engaged *picture* and associated feelings, you are creating the inner environment that matches your success and from which your success oriented action will arise.

ꦩ On a new page in your journal, write "S - See Yourself with Desired Results" as the title at the top. Prepare yourself for this experience by doing the A-B-Cs.

Recall the results you desire for your success with every level of your awareness. What does your desire feel like? Where is your desire? How do you know it from a transient whim or want of ego? To help you discern, *shift* to feeling yourself *want* a piece of chocolate or other tasty temptation.

Notice any differences in how these two states feel. See yourself meet your want of the treat. Enjoy the smells, feel and tastes. What do you gain? How is your life affected by attaining it? What does it inspire? Are you happy? Are you satisfied? How is it valid and rewarding to *want*, attain, and *want* again. But how is that different from living what you truly desire? When have you binged your way to true happiness or struggled your way to relaxation?

Now *shift* to feeling your desire. Imagine being inside yourself, looking through your eyes at your life with this *dream* come true. You are already there...having it, achieving it, sharing it, growing from it, experiencing it...whatever applies.

Notice details, engage your senses, feel your experience of being in your body within that experience. Observe your breathing, facial expressions, and emotions.

How do you think, feel, act, speak? What are your relationships like? How does life flow for you? Dwell in the *real-ity* of what it is like to have what you desired. What *values* do you experience? What do you gain? How is your life affected? Where will this lead you? Are you happy? Are you satisfied?

How is *desire* different from *want* for you? How do you recognize each? Which brings you into the feeling you are seeking? How long does the feeling last? Seeking an object may deliver a shorter term, less satisfying result. The feeling brings energy and will energize, even move you. In general, one comes from an emptiness that seeks to be filled, while the other comes from fullness of soul that seeks expression. This knowledge may help you stay in self-integrity so you are less often misled.

The key to *real-izing* your dream is to evoke it, to actively call it forth through memory and emotionS. Also to invoke it – call upon it – through desire, a powerful force of attraction.

Make notes in your journal. Include surprising details or questions you have or even any blocks and resistances. This visualization may lead you to question what you thought you desired or wanted. In this way it serves as a way to try an idea or satisfy your curiosity vicariously. It is okay to discover something isn't right about it, dispel your illusions, and find it is not what you truly seek. In this case, the next step is to explore that; let it evolve or let it go and choose again.

All of this is valid and valuable information for you. You cannot know every detail with certainty. Consider adding to your intention, "This or something better" to invite and allow for infinite wisdom and possibility.

Recall the experiences of this activity and clarify your thoughts and feelings about your experience Take a few moments to sharpen the vision you desire for yourself, your career, your family life and your future. It's similar to having the lenses flipped during a vision check-up, "Is this clearer or this?" Write what you desire in your journal.

Visualization was a large part of how I realized my dream of living in the Caribbean, and *the feel* was how I recognized the place when I found it. It was also part of how wrote this book for you. Visualization can help you see ways to resolve the root causes of your stress, gain courage and *shift* toward healing. Next, you step into positive action moving forward in the feeling of your success.

CHAPTER 14

STEP INTO POSITIVE ACTION

Florence Nightingale, the Mother of Nursing, said, "I think one's feelings waste themselves in words…" In this book there have been a lot of words used to study the value of unconscious emotions, the related feelings you experience and the energy and information they contain to fuel your success in your work, health and life. You have now arrived at the step in the AH SUCCESS Process that Florence would applaud, because of the balance of what she said about feelings, "…they ought all to be distilled into actions which bring results."

A few fundamental steps or actions that bring results are to simply breathe, shift and let go. These often will soothe, unleash courage or help you become un-stuck until you achieve kinetic expression through more decisive *positive action*. While this step is generally implied to be an outward expression toward your health or other desired outcome, it is truly whatever you are ready, willing and able to do because *shifts* add up to the outcome. Even the most difficult *shifts* can be taken in steps or breaths, each one becoming an accomplishment. Life, from here forward, can be empowering through your steps of choice and will to integrate, express and create.

In the Preface, I mentioned being with you as you step forward into this book, that we would walk through the process together step by step. Whether an emotional step or a physical one, the metaphor is one of walking, taking one step at a time. Even as you step forward on your own afterwards, though we are not standing physically together, hopefully you can perceive that we will continue to be advancing together energetically. Any journey, no matter how far, starts the same...with a step. Having come so far in your learning, you have seen the value of a step-by-step approach yet have gained much in your understanding of manifestation which follows nonlinear quantum principles.

Journal about where you find yourself now compared to where you were as you began the process. With your success in mind, what positive action is before you? Where have you *shifted* and where are you lingering? If you are experiencing hesitation, become aware of what it is about or related to so you can re-frame it. Are you centered? Where do you need to *shift*? Next ask yourself what you need? Do you need to access inner wisdom? Do you need to re-envision your desired results? Just like with the Nursing Process,[1] evaluate and glean any new helpful information, then repeat the AH SUCCESS Process as often as needed integrating any new information each time. The more you feel relief and experience your vibrancy, the more you *real-ize* your success. The more success you express in your life, the more inspiration you give others to do the same.

Step by Step

Each time you take a step (*shift*), it is a new moment, another opportunity to choose. If you feel you missed your mark, you can modify your next step as it arrives. This 'walking through life' in awareness and elevated thinking is a journey. It can sometimes metaphorically feel like taking a step without seeing the staircase, like following a hunch when there is no way to validate it. In the quantum realm, reality is fluid. Everything is 'non-local' until we put energy and intention on it. Just like a quantum particle, it can 'appear' as a result of your intentional inner preparation. This is like manifesting a parking spot or tickets to a sold out concert, or the respiratory therapist showing up a moment before your patient has a seizure and needs airway management. When you see something with your mind's eye and feel it in your heart and body, that is an inner technology of creation and wisdom. You are learning to trust yours. Creating your outer world from this inner world will build the relationship. *Shifting* balances your resiliency and is a sustainable way and means of accomplishment.

There is a type of meditation, a mindfulness-based practice, in which you intentionally focus your thinking on a automatic action such as walking. You carefully observe your experience. You observe the otherwise unnoticed small things that synchronize and connect to make up the grand unified accomplishment such as walking. This practice is more easily done in silence and in a quiet or natural place, but can become second-nature.

Try this walking meditation now. Stand up, center within yourself and begin to step forward. Notice the engagement of any preparatory muscles, including for breathing, prior to any movement of your feet. Observe the progression of weight transfer: a rolling lift of one foot and moving it forward, adjusting it to settle onto the floor with a heel-to-toe sole massaging roll forward. Then transfer your weight while the other foot does a rolling lift, moves forward, adjusts and settles into another roll forward. Notice how your body undulates naturally in a forward wave-like motion. Your arms gracefully swinging in synchronized movements.

As you go through these phases of this activity, notice the balance of your head on your shoulders, your breath, and any tension or restriction that limits the fluidity in the motion. Your mind may wander, so notice when it drifts and bring it back each time to observe the experience of walking. This practice can be 15-30 minutes in your hallway or in the yard. Try it barefoot, especially if you can do so on grass or bare earth.

As you become accustomed to observing yourself while in motion, you can bring this enjoyable practice into your everyday activities. The intent is to experience full aware-ness and presence, especially during autopilot activities, where you lose valuable time and experience of your life by staying connected to the whirl and rush or gloom and stress. Your mind become empty of the flurry of thought and stress and full of awareness and wonder.

Walking Toward Success

Walking toward a goal is more often a process with a trajectory rather than a step-over-the-line and into-your-dream moment.

> For many years prior to moving to the Caribbean, I'd say, "My body may be here, but my heart is in the Caribbean." That was a quantum statement. I knew where I was standing physi-cally and it was different from where I wanted to be. It seemed that only a miracle could bridge the disparity, because I did not know how to make it happen. I listened to island music that made me feel like I was there and splashed the sun-soaked pastel colors in the decor of my home. I had a *picture* of the white sand beach and crystal blue water in my mind and on my clipboard at work. I wore flowery, colorful clothing and believed every step I was taking in life led to my dream.
>
> It was illogical to think that when I went west from Florida to work as a traveling nurse in Texas, California and Hawaii that I would end up southeast in the Caribbean. Yet I felt a deep calm about living in the Caribbean one day. I spoke of it happening just as one would talk about plans for their birthday. That *shift* in perception, *to hold space* for positive possibility was the miracle it took. That state of mind was the link to my des-tiny and the steps to it appeared as I became ready to take them.

Because of the connectedness of all things, something magic hap-pens in the manifestation of health, success or a dream. Its *real-ization* happens both forward and backward. Your active desire and centered knowing resonate with the dream and draw it to you while the dream draws you to it, no matter what odd turns you to take. Positive action is not always on a direct path as there are many paths.

When you are fully engaged in something, become unaware of *doing* and are fully present in being – even for just a few moments – time expands and you have a richer experience. Your breathing slows, the vagus nerve is stimulated, your thoughts give way to wonder, your heart radiates an attractive strong emotion and you fully enjoy the moment. Do you realize that this is a health-producing state? It is also a neurochemical state similar to falling in love that boosts immunity and seems to warp time.

> Bring to mind a time of infatuation, immersion or falling in love – when you felt the timelessness of being fully engaged. Maybe you got lost in a creative project, admiring your baby or present with a patient's story. Engage with your recollection and experience it now. How did it feel? Were you so immersed that you didn't feel your body or experience time? Describe the state you were in and your world of awareness in that experience. Maybe you felt a magnetism, a connection, a lack of separation, or *no thing?* Journal about the qualities of your experience. Note what cues tell you you're in this state.

When you are so engaged that you lose track of place, time, even self, you experience pure consciousness. Your body is governed by vagal influence and an associated neurochemical broth. You can observe this state with awareness, without judgement. The moment you realize your experience and name it with your mind, you are jolted back into the space-time reality of your normal consciousness. Notice as this *shift* happens for you. Notice the change in your physiology by way of breathing, heart rate, body temperature, mental alertness and awareness. If you can reflect upon *where you were,* then *where are you* in the current moment while doing the reflecting? This is the difference between *no where* and *now here*. Athletes, artists, new mothers, and people healing from disease find this state known as 'flow' or 'being in the zone' to be a blessing and a marvel. You can learn to dwell there. The A-B-Cs can help create the parasympathetic dominant milieu in your body and meditation can lead to the expansive state of consciousness. With practice you can *shift* at will.

Being fully present is different from many experiences you have on the job, especially time-bound productivity and multi-tasking. Research has proven that you cannot multi-task; you are actually just switching your focus quickly. Mastering those moments with presence and honing your ability to *shift* are essential. Slowing down and even single-tasking may be a future innovative adaptation for your job. You have already felt stress related to this as your job tasks and related knowledge have accelerated in complexity, while changes in practice and work flows have become the norm. Ongoing stress can surpass building agility, to dull cognition and cause reduced mental sharpness. Also as unfamiliarity with and the complexity of tasks increase, time efficiency is lost.[2] The bottom line is multitasking usually leads to less productivity and more mistakes.[3]

Re-member Your Heart

Stress can make you feel *dis-membered*, pulled apart, separate from what you love. One antidote to the isolation of fight-or-flight is to join, connect or re-member. When disconnected from your co-workers, your dream, your family or your self, work through the steps of the Process with whatever is calling you to re-member and re-connect to your heart, health and purpose.

Everything you do is accomplished with small steps, from getting ready for work to doing a treatment procedure. Having your heart aligned with your purpose and goal is like an autopilot that maintains your course, adjusting for wave fluctuations, currents and wind. It magnetizes your outcome and can improve your tolerance and resilience around stress. On the hand, the physiology of stress is damaging to health when it overwhelms your ability to adapt and re-stabilize.[4]

Step into Communication

Learning to speak and communicate to bring your wisdom and ideas out for consideration, and to influence a new paradigm for the well-being of your community may be a new positive action for a nurse.

You and I know nurses can be competitive, jealous, gossipy, back-stabbing, perfectionistic, even controlling. We can recognize the verbal and body language of a colleague acting as a martyr, demonstrating their effort and frustration by speaking in terms of 'never' and 'always' – even declining help and doing it herself 'as usual'.

Communication and asking for what you need are skills to develop and hone by using the Process to get clear and in touch with the heart of the matter. You will feel empowered and eventually find you have more influence by communicating more coherently. Communication and managing your emotions, even stress, are high determinants of success, often over knowledge and education.

Step into Emotional Intelligence

When nurses don't like something or feel something is wrong, do they suck it up, speak with a colleague for validation or gossip with others to build an us-versus-them mentality? Might they whine or complain at a staff meeting if something is getting bad enough? If nurses stew long enough, anger brews and they may spew an opinion or two. But, honestly, who listens to anyone who comes from the low vibratory state of a victim? When you talk optimistically or empowered, you might initially get the who-are-you or what-makes-you-different attitude from colleagues or your manager.

There is a pecking order established when people work together in *co-operation* toward a goal, including among nurses. This is different from co-creation which involves an elevation in premise. To elevate your thinking to *co-creation*, can shake up that leader-follower hierarchy and, though unintended, can cause a shake-up. Often this is when a colleague will leave their job or place of employment because their urge for creativity reveals they have outgrown their position or the group consciousness required to stay in the rut.

Remember Rachel who had the amygdala hijack at work? Soon after, she took positive action, moved onward and upward in her career to a private perinatal service center and management opportunities that were less likely to have been available in her former workplace. Never having debriefed from the incident with Rachel, nor given any reinforcement for her skill or behavior modification, her manager's profound depart-ing words were, "I knew you'd outgrow us quickly." Rachel's soul was speaking loudly to her the day of the hijack. She was in deep resistance because she had ignored the early signals and was being pushed by her work situation to grow.

Be *response-able* for the way you feel. Doing so will help you com-municate more clearly. You become more *able to respond* rather than react as you more accurately discern your choices and choose your ac-tions. By separating your personal emotion from an encounter or com-munication, you avoid tainting the essence of your effort and message.

Step into Empowerment

Whether you take positive steps toward your dream – or toward breaking out of any subliminal patterns not serving of yourself, col-leagues and patients – you triumph. These 'stuck-patterns' are of an insecurity, scarcity and fear-based mindset. They seed stress and illness. Having a voice, speaking, and communicating are not about the yang of fighting, which is not the outward preference of a nurse, but rather the yin of changing from within and communicating from heart and wholeness.

Anger is a symptom, a messenger, even when justified. There is something needing attention or expression. When anger is the fuel for change, all the quantum principles still apply, so be careful. It is a good time pause and start back at step one with awareness, to differentiate your emotions and actions from that of a tantrum. Seek to discover the seed thought that flanked your perspective. You want to manifest con-sciously. No matter the circumstance, there is a lesson and therein lies empowerment for you. If you realize it and open to hold the space for a new possibility, you can *shift* to choice from victim using inner wisdom and bring the momentum of the change into alignment with your true intentional purpose. Empowerment is not about *speaking* your truth from wounds, but *seeking* truth and acting from within it. This integrity sources the power.

Step into Influence

The power of influence comes more from how you do something than what you do or what you teach. Nurses have lots of knowledge and, with the benefits from self-care, are empowered with what it takes to be influential in any area they choose.

You know how every department makes changes to suit their work-flow, and it all rolls down to the nurses to dovetail the compartmental-ized decisions at the interface with the patient. The other departments and managers depend upon you to figure it out, and they know you will, but will they listen to you?

The amazing plate spinner on a 1969 episode of *The Ed Sullivan Show* comes to mind.[5] Look it up online and see if it doesn't remind you of your job. You will laugh because, like the spinner, you make it look easy. While protecting the patient from the reality of things that just don't work, you know when you're putting your job on the line.

You are a synthesizer of information, situations, circumstances and human responses, along with policies, procedures, practice standards and customary unit protocols. You can crystallize what needs to happen, and achieve it safely with a smile and heart. Nurses, as synthesizers, are instrumental to moving forward in caring for health.

The ideas and solutions of nurses have merit and are worth listening to, considering and integrating. As you step forward, building your abilities in communication, including assertiveness skills will help you take step after step. Action by speaking with clarity is important to help the public, health providers, employers, policy makers and colleagues understand what nurses do and need to accomplish their jobs. Traditionally, nurses have a 'yes' role in their jobs, doing anything instructed and anything that is necessary. Another part of success, as you walk into empowerment and become more influential, is the ability to use one skill that Warren Buffett says "separates really successful people from everyone else... saying no..."[6] This comprises having boundaries for yourself, deciding and choosing from your top priority goals what gets your time and attention, and not working to the detriment of personal and family time, but rather toward and elevated life and health. It is also important for your family, who depends upon you to 'always be there,' to understand and learn to walk for themselves. This creates health within your family.

Learn to say no with love.

Step into Joy

Happiness is periodic, situational, and comes and goes. It is reason dependent and pleasing. A unique thing about happiness is that we can intentionally pursue it and also manufacture it through visualization and the neurochemistry of our brain. Here are a couple of my secrets to happiness:

1. Aim high, so if you fall short you are still delighted and successful.
2. Consider having at least three dreams at all times: One dream you are realizing in the present; one that you are working on; and another just in case one falls through.

Joy is different. It arises from an internal source. It endures, warms and promotes contentment. As a yin characteristic, it balances stress and empowers you. Joy emanates from your inner values, virtues and wholeness, and shines upon your journey despite the external conditions.

As you walk the AH SUCCESS path of integrity with yourself, joy cannot help but spill into and influence your life, choices, circumstance and relationships. Give permission to yourself to experience happiness and express joy. If you have been suffering from stress, it may have stunted your brain and blunted your feelings of spontaneity, creativity, self-acceptance, happiness or joy. As you release and relax, accept and embrace, these things will bubble up and flow into expression. Then you will realize that you are still standing and breathing, and it becomes okay for the real, healthy you to emerge and express. Your patients will love it. They will feel they are receiving safer, quality care from an empowered nurse.

Integration

You may have a job that meets your lower level Maslow hierarchy-type needs, but what are you creating within the inner environment of your body and life that resonates with your soul and health? When your thoughts, feelings and actions are in alignment with your purpose, your *real-ity* mirrors to you the results of that vibration, even during tough times.

(Ⓢ) On a new page in your journal, write "S - Step into Positive Action" as the title at the top. Prepare yourself for this experience by doing the A-B-Cs.

Recall your picture of success and experience it now. From this feeling, this state of success, feel your current self drawn to this experience. Let the feelings magnetize you to attract your success. Feel the pull, draw and yearn for your success. Elevate to match the vibration and feeling of your success. Notice how things shift in resonance. Anything out of resonance dissipates, moves aside, and is a non-issue as you stay focused on and in resonance with your success.

See yourself walking in your success, taking steps while stepping stones and paths form before you. Let the imagery spontaneously occur as you keep moving forward, step by step. You do not have to know what these steps are, just embody the vibration and trust it will be matched as the steps, mentors, opportunities and lessons appear with purposeful timing.

Some steps toward your success are tangible and logical. List any that come to you so you can take positive actions on them. The many steps that are unseen, intangible, internal and immeasurable by any scientific equipment available are the most powerful. These are what change your health, perception, situation, *real-ity*, hence your life. They establish and hold the resonant vibration. Let your positive actions be guided by this essence which lets you recognize success for yourself.

Fully embody your success – the happiness and joy from cultivating, creating and striving. Pay attention to your feelings and emotions, and the multiple ways success is communicated to you. Do you feel light, expanded, warm, grounded, liquid, boundless, satiated or joyful? Choose to do things that create feelings of success for you. Allow yourself to create this soulful state, every morning for 5 minutes minimum, and be in it several times a day, the longer and more frequent, the better.

Take this brief amount of time for yourself daily to build momentum and transform. Use your journal to record the lists, prompts and inspirations from this activity. Feel gratitude for this rich inner wisdom.

This is how I knew when I found my home in the Caribbean. Then, while arriving by ferry boat into the little island harbor the first time, tears welled in my eyes as my soul became enlivened. I looked around and said what I felt, "I am home." Expression of Soul makes us feel like our true self, or like we're home. Though I'd never seen this paradise before, I recognized its nature and beauty by way of the resonant vitality I felt within myself. I had arrived home and there my soul still dwells.

Years later, I followed my heart, in love, to California but the culture-change to living stateside was shocking. When the weight of a stressful and toxic work-environment began to feel less like success for me, it was time to grow. Again, using these principles and techniques, I made my way to the creation of the manuscript for this book and the AH SUCCESS Process.

A purpose of all life is growth. From whereever you are in your journey, repeat the steps of the AH SUCCESS Process to clarify, deepen, expand or modify your experience as you grow, create and move forward.

PART THREE

EMPOWERMENT & INFLUENCE

Transformation inherently arises from what has been. Use your stress for positive change.

Because you possess mastery of your job, want to contribute more and make a larger difference, it is not surprising that you found yourself at a point of awareness, challenge and transformation — the jeopardy of your own well-being. By taming the effects of your stress you will see things differently and find you have the courage to be creative, influence change, build community and cultivate wholism.

Can you see that you are taking part in a modern-day version of the mythological Hero's Journey?

Are you aware that there is something strongly favoring your success, empowerment and influence? — an environment. Combined with your inner milieu, readiness and ability, many eternal factors and variables today contribute to it and present timely opportunities to entertain alternative possibilities for yourself, your health and your career. This phenomenon called "kairos" refers to a time when the conditions are right for accomplishing a crucial action — when it's the opportune and decisive moment.

Part Three covers how to thrive beyond potential obstacles you may face on your journey from stress to success. It looks into the elements of the current kairos, and helps you realize, the true influential power is not control, but inspiration.

CHAPTER 15

OVERCOMING OBSTACLES

Obstacles are inevitable in life and on the way to success. On this sometimes rough terrain, many *germs* like *attitudin-algia* and *excuse-itis* are lurking and ready to take advantage of any weakened awareness, loss of focus or stressed sense of self. The A-B-Cs will help you face and overcome them on your way through the steps to AH SUCCESS. Living from your center, shines *antimicrobial* light on obstacles and challenges. They become messengers. If you look at them as an opportunity for growth, it makes the prize sweeter.

Knowledge of yourself – deep and honest awareness and wisdom of your intentions, aspirations, blocks and barriers – will always be a fine companion as you journey forward. Learning about common obstacles you may encounter as you make *shifts*, choose differently, take care of yourself, and move forward will help you reduce potential stress and discern your *response-ability*.

Perhaps you can already feel incremental or dimensional changes for yourself since you first noticed your inner call light. You've had many experiences since then. Not only do we change because of our experiences, experience changes us; it molds, shapes, rebuilds, heals, polishes and opens. There may be subtle but powerful changes within your perception, the magnetics of which will bring about change in more tangible ways. As things are revealed, new neural pathways are reinforced through your awareness. Living from a new perspective means expressing it in your life through your choices – how you speak, act, feed your body and contribute to the ecology of nature.

What have you learned about your self, your stress, your challenges and opportunities? Make notes in your journal about how your awareness has changed or been reinforced. How do you feel now? What do you see yourself doing differently? How will you continue to nurture your successes?

In your journal make a list of situations and issues you wish to have success around. Next to each write how it feels to have each success for you. This is your awareness list. Each of these provide a basis to journey through the AH SUCCESS Process. Each feeling is a guide inward toward your inner wisdom. Any feeling that moves outward as an emotion and dominates your personality will obscure your true self, so be careful.

As you work with your list, you may find that you move through some more quickly as there are crosslinked connections of truth and wisdom between issues, challenges and visions. In this way, the healing of a single dilemma can facilitate the healing of many; it resembles a process of purification.

When you feel successful and have a new perspective, there are common lessons, issues and obstacles you may encounter as you move forward. It may seem that you are more sensitive as you seek resonance between the *real-ities* of your inner and outer worlds, and as you go from your personal life into your work life. Especially in the beginning of implementing the Process, seeing things differently can seem confusing, frustrating or dismaying. Take the time to be in stillness, saturating your being with feelings of your success. Do the A-B-Cs in the moment and work through the AH SUCCESS Process with anything that needs self reflection, deeper understanding and transformation. Make notes in your journal about your experiences and personal wisdoms from working through the Process.

Overcome Feeling Fear

Have you become open to creating your reality? Henry Ford is attributed with saying, "Whether you believe you can or cannot, you are correct."[1] Perceptions and feelings are part of the epigenetics of the expression of genes and events in life.

Fear is an emotion that intensely affects your physiology, shunting blood supply from the frontal cortex and releasing excitatory hormones that draw heavily on the energy resources in your body. If fear is warranted in your situation, do what you need to do to be safe and seek help. But often fear *feels* justified when it has no real substance. In this case, you can think of fear as "false evidence appearing real." It can arise from an internal story, belief or other bad experience we believe has power at that moment. Ask yourself, *"Is this situation truly a matter to react to as if it were life or death?"* or *"Am I remembering, imaging or is this actually happening to me now?"* Go within and discern what is true.

When the brain detects a change, it naturally defaults to protect. This reactionary and habitual response is effective in the interest of efficiency and survival. The brain is wired to reject pain, including the pain of making personal changes. Awareness of this is important to your success. Do the A-B-Cs to recognize, feel and move beyond that protective physiology when it is digressive. From your center, create health-supporting physiology and reinforce neural connections that support positive emotions, success and well-being.

Venturing to operate while maintaining this neuro-physiology can be challenging as new and familiar situations may cause anxiety. Staying centered allows a stabilizing fulcrum for emotions and a clarifying filter for discerning any seeds of fear that may be sprout within.

Just before Luke Skywalker enters into the Cave of Evil on the planet of Dagobah in the Star Wars film, *The Empire Strikes Back*, Luke asks Yoda, "What is in the cave?" Yoda answers, "Only what you take with you."[2] You may or may not recall that Luke brought his lightsaber and indeed met Darth Vader inside the cave. They dueled and he beheaded Darth Vader with his weapon. When Luke peered into Darth Vader's helmet, it was his own face that it contained. For Luke, it was a metaphorical journey of facing his inner fears. For some, the cave may represent the discernment of what is real and what is false. Think about what it represents for you. What expresses from your subconscious in situations and life in general, and how is it working for you?

Think of one courageous act by you or another person. Was it done despite risk and while overcoming fear? Fear is always present in acts of courage. Fear and courage are seemingly opposite emotions. But more accurately, they are in relationship like that of Yin and Yang. They co-exist, yet the seed to transform each lies within the other. One crescendoes into a expression over the other and then recedes once again into a dynamic surging balance.

> ♥ What do you fear in relation to your success? What situations, people or decisions cause you fear? Which of your own characteristics do you fear? Write these in your journal in a column on the left side of a page. Write beside each, in a column on the right side, a balancing characteristic of yourself.
>
> Pause and take a moment to experience each of those affirmative characteristics, individually feeling them fully in your body. Then feel in your *body* and *being* how one *shifts* into the other as you move between them. Perhaps visualizing yourself in a fearful circumstance and the *shifting* into courage within that or another situation would be helpful. Inquire more deeply by working through the AH SUCCESS Process with each of the situations, people or decisions you have written down as part of this Heart Activity.

Overcome Feeling Alone

In the Winnie the Pooh stories, there is a bouncing tiger named Tigger, who happily says, "…I'm the only one."[3] However, while he is elated thinking that being unique is a wonderful thing, you may feel lonely and alone in your endeavor to raise your vibration and live in health if you are feeling a lack of support or community. Have you ever started doing something for yourself and met with resistance or inertia from your family? It remains up to you to be accountable to yourself and your decision. Only you can set aside the time and define its use.

(♥) Make notes of your common blocks and challenges to having time to yourself and for your self care. Being aware of them will be helpful in planning how to face, adjust or otherwise handle them when they present.

Solitude has a balancing place in life, especially the busy and stressful life of a nurse. This is time of respite and renewal, creativity and regeneration. But be aware, isolation can indicate that there is more ego involved than you realize. When this occurs, the ego is doing what it does well – blocking and separating, which is not the same as healing from solitude. Remember, healing is about becoming whole. Use the steps in the Process to embrace and bless your ego. Listen for any deeper message or meaning.

Look for beauty in the light let in by the crack and reach out. Go within and connect with your inner wisdom that is deeper than those isolating thoughts. Find connection by centering deeply within your heart. If you have young children, they are terrific teachers. Watch them to observe wonder and animation of pure life energy – and listen to their laughter, bubbling up in joy. Model this to enjoy it with them and magnify it for yourself.

Respect the rules of your job, but better yourself and hold your intention as you influence a healthier, more unified culture. Despite acting independently at first, you will reach out in health to build supportive and influential relationships with your colleagues, friends and family. Meet your patients with your heart and you will both move from being *alone* to *all one*.

Overcome Feeling Doubt

This is when you meet the 'committee in your head' that seems to second guess everything you think or do. Some voices may be familiar subconscious programs that you examined in Chapter 7. The committee will find many chances to rally as you move from stress to success. Maybe you have previously been able to ignore them by engaging in some mindless activity like video games or watching TV to cope. Perhaps you squelch their voices by devouring a bag of cookies or having some wine. Now you can develop positively affirmative behaviors. Dispelling doubt through accomplishment can be as simple as getting up and going for a walk.

> What have you used to distract yourself from your intentions and goals? How have you drown out voices of doubt? Ask yourself if any of these interventions ever had any lasting positive effect beyond any momentary feeling. What feeling did you achieve from each? If it is gratifying, be still and let that feeling sink in, becoming aware of how it feels in your body. You experience feelings because of the movement of energy. This movement can build into the momentum necessary for a *shift*, then transform into the energy of positive action. Seek experiences that feel like confidence, clarity, sincerity or whatever is a desirable feeling for you. Note in your journal any prompts to help you get back on track when needed.
>
> You might also get unsolicited feedback from others who feel entitled to prune your growth with words from their limiting beliefs and programming, such as:

» You seem different.

» You never used to...

» You should...

» Oh, so suddenly you have time to......?

» What's wrong with you?

» Maybe you should...

In a column going down the left side of the page in your journal, list the above and other examples of this type of feedback that you have received from others in response to a change in behavior resulting from a new choice you made. Next, across from each one, write your positive statement of truth. The comment "You seem different" may become an empowering self-truth such as "I am growing".

Have one or more positive statements of truth for each feedback item you have listed. Also consider writing these positive self-truths on 3x5 cards and decorate them to make them fun and motivating. Then pick one for daily or in-the-moment affirmative inspiration.

If you are acting from your values, therein lies the intrinsic power to forgive these potential saboteurs and to dispel doubt. This is how self integrity is established so you can live healthy and happily with yourself rather than depending on outside approval. When you are *real-izing* the benefits, such as sleeping better, having more energy or more tolerance, and feeling happier or otherwise empowered, others will soon be eager to know what new thing you are doing. Misery does love company, but everyone truly seeks to feel healthy and happy, so they will want some of what you have.

Overcome Feeling Overwhelmed

At times, you may feel you have hit a wall that seems impenetrable. You may feel lost or like you are going backwards, maybe even hopeless or angry. Perhaps you may feel as if all is bigger than you and you doubt that whatever you can do will matter. Just stop. Realize that you were granted another breath. This new moment presents an opening for new possibilities. Realize that it is just how you are feeling and that it can pass like a rain cloud. You have much in your favor, despite seeming stuck at times. You can *shift* that physiology with the A-B-Cs. Practice building your intuitive heart-brain connection with the skills of the AH

SUCCESS Process.

"Remember, you are not going back, you are moving forward!" I give you these words of encouragement, as I did my clients who expressed dread for going "back to the states" near the end of their island retreat vacations. They had come to know something very valuable while on-island, something many were not aware of... knowledge of themselves feeling healthy and happy.[4] You have similar inner knowledge while nearing a similar rite of passage of your own. I suggest for you, as I did then, to choose a word or picture in your mind for how you feel when at ease, empowered, clear and heart-centered. Recall it as needed to refresh your experience of health and joy. Practice until you know the experience as yourself rather than as an effect and live from that truth.

This is not the path of least resistance. You must maintain self reliance, trust and commitment because much of the resistance is actually within yourself. Overcoming it will provide you a more profound inner strength and empowerment.

The way to progress – rather than resist – is to cultivate what you want including the thoughts and feelings. As I learned from research done by the HeartMath Institute, use the power of your heart-based feelings you associate with your achievement to internalize the power of their effect. The feeling of empowerment is within you and not in an external source,

Start within yourself. Do the A-B-Cs and grow from there through the AH SUCCESS Process. Growth is what you are called to do, because you are alive. Growth in this way is not linear, it is multidimensional. This can propel your advancement by many steps like when a rubber band is stretched backward and then dramatically lunges forward when released. It is a process of moving forward, so carry on from wherever you are now with the new information and create new positive associations and neural pathways as you grow.

Continue learning and be open to a new desirable future of well-being and the new scientific research that supports these principles. Joe Dispenza encourages, "...learn to think greater than your feelings."[5] Your mind is naturally creative. Necessity births solutions and innovations through creativity.

As you use what you have been learning to walk toward your power and success, it is possible that you may still have feelings of powerlessness. How do you experience powerlessness? What situations, circumstances, interactions, people or thoughts make you feel powerless? List them in your journal, then prioritize by importance or impact. Over time, explore them individually using the AH SUCCESS Process. Elevate, get the lessons, and make those lessons into tools for your success. What cues can you glean, especially thoughts and feelings that you have, to warn you of situations or circumstances where powerlessness might still loom for you? Use this awareness to transform these opportunities into success. Also note these in your journal.

Overcome Feeling Confused

Going through change can seem turbulent and confusing. As you do one thing differently, there may be a domino or prismatic effect within your emotions and life as they are *entangled* with one another. This can also be exciting because it is evidence of your vision gaining traction. When you hold your dream or picture close, it becomes an element of influence for your decisions, choices, actions and even relationships. Increasing the coherence in your mind, body and actions becomes an electromagnetic force of attraction within your life. It then becomes a part of your still and quiet center where your truth lies.

In contrast, the noise of the world, your job or fears can become louder, tugging and pushing you back toward the depths you are emerging from. Facing and overcoming these challenges are likely part of the alchemy to reorder and shape your success.

Meditation will help you heal and stay centered. You will need to draw upon your resilience to weather the storm, so keep doing the A-B-Cs in the moment and sustain the feeling in your heart. Pace yourself. In this way too, you are creating new neural pathways, chemical-hormonal sequences, emotional responses and magnetic resonances to support your well-being and success.

At times of enthusiasm, you will want to share your new discoveries with the world. Be cautious. Doing so in a haphazard manner may create turbulence which can lead to confusion. This relates to another lesson from my island life to share with you.

The crystal blue waters in the Caribbean are known for deep visibility, wondrous colorful fish and amazing reefs. Yet some visitors obscure the beauty before them in their scurry to see it. They will emerge after a swim, in dismay, reporting that the water was murky , there was nothing to see, and there were no fish. What they did not know is that there is a way to be with nature, to avoid clashing with that environment. The clouded water is evidence. There is a way to enter the water that allows you to observe. One must become still and relaxed to avoid stirring the sand. If it is disturbed, be patient. Become present with the settling of the sand and feel yourself settle with it. One needs to be calm and centered because the fish will stay around or eventually reappear if they sense harmony rather than fear.

Returning to the States from the Caribbean, to work from vacation or to your routine *life* with new knowledge from a convention or doing the Process requires patience and tolerance. Preaching your new methods or demanding that others listen will likely deafen them. Trying harder can be like flailing in futility to see the fish only to cloud the water and chase them away. Often it can be less about doing and more about being. Become still and certain of what you know in your heart, to feel through and beyond the confusion in your mind. Change is not always pretty, but it can contain grace none the less. Cultivate your vitality within and the murkiness will clear and some recognizable and desirable qualities will appear as did the fish.

⌇ What things are confusing for you about your stress, job or life? In what way do you find them confusing? List these in your journal pairing them with any distinct desired characteristics you need or wish to express in relation to them.

Use the AH SUCCESS Process to help sort things out.

Ask empowering questions, such as, "What can I let go of that is no longer serving me?" or "What differences do I feel in myself when I feel {*this way*}?" Record your answers. Seek to understand, *Why is this happening to me?* By exploring the answers to questions like "What do I need to learn?" or "What is trying to express through me?" or "What am I holding onto, overlooking or have yet to accept?"

Alternatively, fill in the blanks in this sentence:

I could see _____ instead of _____ .

This is based upon lessons from *A Course In Miracles*. For example, "I could see that I have choices" instead of "I am stuck in this job." Try completing this sentence several times until you find what resonates as true for you. Be reassured – wholeness is not about being cookie-cutter perfect. It is about acknowledging and working with all that is.

Overcome Feeling Stuck

You may be asking how you can be so successful by numerous benchmarks coveted by society, but still feel stuck? It may be helpful to review some of your journal notes from the Heart Activities about your thoughts, habits, desires and wisdoms. You could be following habitual "shoulds" and working toward goals that don't actually align with who you are or what you truly want. Mindset and Performance Coach, Dr. Kerry Petsinger calls these "False Objectives".[6]

Feeling stuck can arise when caught in *paradox*. Sometimes things are not as they appear. Logical outcomes can seem contradictory, ends do not meet and more questions appear. You may be working harder but accomplish less, improve your efficiency but still not have enough time, or do more but continue to get marginal outcomes. This can be frustrating and confusing, but this is *paradox*.

It can be difficult to accept that not everything will go exactly the way you want, when you want even when you do the A-B-Cs or the AH SUCCESS Process. The rewards may not come on a one-to-one return. It may seem like you are going backwards or like nothing is happening at all, then suddenly things can turn towards a positive .

As for handling your stress, the practice of self-regulation takes on-going effort. Building and sustaining coherence is worth it. Life without it is frustrating and depleting.

There are disparities that are arise from the dovetailing of philoso-phies, rules, cultures and values that we can recognize as paradoxical. For example, how you can be expected to accept another patient when you haven't had a break yet. Paradox differs from the conflicts and power struggles that may develop because of paradox. Paradox needs to be given space and allowed room for possibility. This is because of the interrelatedness of things and a holistic perspective, which by its nature, allows for diversity. In this paradigm, something new can be expressed from the dynamic. This can explain how, when you endeavor to change, things can paradoxically seem to get more difficult and messier. This seems to be life's way of testing your clarity and commitment. Use your *stick-to-it-ness* for your own well-being.

It is an all too common paradox for seemingly successful people, who appear to have it all, to feel stuck. Authenticity is often an under-lying issue. The AH SUCCESS Process assists you with becoming an honest friend to yourself and creating ways to live a healthy coherent life. Moving from stress to success begs for authenticity.

> Are there places where you feel stuck? Where do you feel stuck? What is keeping your stuck? Consider things like, "I can always find time to drive the children to another activity, but cannot find time for myself to meditate." What 'false objectives' have become apparent to you? Do you truly want to heal, to have success? What seems to be lost with success? Write your answers and responses in your journal as you consider these ideas.
>
> Also note in your journal where have you experienced paradox in your life. Contemplate each for messages and

messengers. What new information and understanding can you gain? Review how you handled the paradox or messages and what you can do differently now. List these lessons, tactics and skills in your journal. As you move forward you may be challenged by what appear to be obstacles that may paradoxically be stepping stones. These can be valuable insights and lessons to keep handy and refer to when you need inspiration and understanding. Do add them to your journal as you glean more wisdom.

A-B-C for AH SUCCESS

If you cannot reason, or if stress is too much, use the Easy as A-B-C Technique. If you need reassurance or clarity, do the A-B-Cs. It is a simple tool for *in-the-moment* self regulation which is the basis of the AH SUCCESS Process. This allows you to shift your physiology and thoughts to heart-felt safety, ease and care. Remember, healing is a process that cannot occur in flight-or-flight. Reliance is cultivated from shifting. Desired change is also a process. To go deeper toward success, work through the Process time and time again. You may want to refer to the list in Chapter 4 of your feelings associated with your *desired state*. Continue to work through the Process until you enjoy feeling the feelings of your desired states of relaxation and resilience. Then continue until you are expressing them joyfully, freely and creatively in your life.

After you gain experience and connection with the skills, you'll naturally model your embodied knowledge. Consider teaching the basics to an interested colleague, your partner or child. It's helpful to have those around you be *response-able*, tend to their self care, and elevate their thinking too. It can improve communication, relationships and health. Suggest this book to a friend or colleague so you can share the learning and build your healthy community.

Keep in mind that your experience is about you and their experience is about them. Theirs may be different and though concepts may be universal, meanings and lessons can be very personal and are found within. If you get stuck or face any obstacle, use the AH SUCCESS Process to see the paradox and beyond into your authentic objectives and holistic purpose.

Three Paradoxes

It will be helpful to be aware of and contemplate the following:

What you want to see in the world, create in yourself first.
If you resonate with the information you glean, if it improves your life and inspires you toward health, then use it to do just that. In doing so for yourself, you will serve the world.

The 'true you' is a conscious essence that is unchangeable.
It's your perceptions and reactions that change, which influences that which changes your world. This is explained by the words of author Joyce Carol Oates from Solstice. Say this to yourself as your read her words, "I never change, I simply become more myself."8 We have talked about changing your behaviors, neuro-physiology, perceptions and thoughts, but the truth of your being is changeless and awaiting reveal-ation (revelation).

You never truly seek to have the thing, the job, the relation-ship or to accomplish the goal.
What you truly seek is to feel the way that you perceive you would feel if you had it. So create and experience that feeling and let it be your guide.

Contemplate the three paradoxes and make notes in your journal about your musing and discoveries. Next, consider what life, the world and your work unit would look and feel like with happy, calm, creative, resilient, empowered, influential...

...you? ...nurses? ...patients?

In your journal, make a two-page spread. Your will create three columns for this exercise. As you consider these, write about your vision for each in your journal. List goals, aspirations and wants in the left column. You may want to lose weight, stay in your current job to retain seniority, get a promotion, buy a new car, get veneers put on your teeth or purchase a new house. Next, in the middle column, list beside each why you want that or what having that thing will mean for you. Examples are: because I will get more vacation time, a raise, a partner, better gas mileage, whiter teeth or because I deserve it. In the third column, on the right side, write how you will feel when you have that which you seek. Examples may be, I will feel free, loved, like a part of the solution, confident, safe and comfortable. Take time to feel each of these feelings within your body. The experience of these desired feelings are an important part of how you will know and have success.

As you move forward, keep the result (the feeling) in mind and act from the empowerment of your vision and feelings to guide you toward the highest expression of your self. That is truly your reason, inspiration and success.

CHAPTER 16

DARE TO MAKE A DIFFERENCE

Women and nurses who have insight around the plights and challenges of their jobs, work environment, care of others, and their own needs often find they must keep their thoughts to themselves, stay in line and not interrupt the flow of the yang-ness of a system.

"Seldom do nurses get interviewed and quoted."[1] This phenomenon and details were noticed, researched and revealed by journalists, Bernice Buresh and Suzanne Gordon in their book, *From Silence to Voice: What Nurses Know and Must Communicate to the Public*. They fully support nurses giving a voice to what they do, and they know it takes courage to do this.

If your experience of stress takes you to the point of near-exhaustion or more serious symptoms, you and I both know you do not physically or emotionally burn out after one or two incidents of stress. If the results, feedback, merit or reward on the job rarely meet your true needs, goals and wants, you may feel unfulfilled personally and invalidated professionally. This gradual and cyclical process can lead, over time, to lower energy, motivation and satisfaction and – most sadly – less compassion and health. Tim McClure, executive coach, author and speaker suggests, "The biggest concern of any organization should be when its most passionate people become quiet."[2] But organizations tend to prefer quiet conformity. *Your* ache, longing and quiet contains power which can create or destroy, depending upon what you cultivate.

To successfully make a difference from your quietness, solitude and truth is different from an assertion or domination. As you learn to make a difference from the strength of your self knowledge, self care and compassion – yang traits will show up because they seem to be *the way* in the world, business, and healthcare. For inspiration on this, listen to *the invitation message* in this except from the beautiful prose-poem by that name.

> It doesn't interest me what you do for a living. I want to know what you ache for, and if you dare to dream of meeting
>
> your heart's longing...
>
> I want to know if you can see beauty even when it's not pretty, every day, and if you can source your own life from its
>
> presence...
>
> I want to know
>
> if you can be alone with yourself and if you truly like the company you keep in the empty moments.
>
> — *an excerpt from Oriah "Mountain Dreamer" House's prose-poem, "The Invitation."*[3]

Can you begin to see beauty in imperfection – the crack, the light, the possibility, the opportunity? Can you now be alone with yourself, sitting quietly, in peaceful company with the things that contribute to your job and health stress, along with your resistance to or incongruence with them? Are you gaining an elevated perspective of your quiet and fatigue as a calling rather than a desperate futility? Will you let go, forgive and listen with compassion for the whispers? The *way* is through. Continue to journal as a way to explore your wondrous self. Continue to cultivate awareness, resiliency, creativity and community because of the value for yourself and your colleagues.

Though the pressures seem to be from the outside, the pressure is within you, acting as a messenger to serve you and your purpose. To aim outward at them is to spur a revolution. To answer your inner call light and go within is to influence an evolution. "Your playing small doesn't serve the world" according to Marianne Williamson in her beautiful prose-poem, *Our Deepest Fear*.[4] You are a nurse, an advocate, a facilitator, a caregiver, a healer, and you are an amazing and powerful being. You are called to your career in service. You are being called to grow. A healer's ability to facilitate healing in others is only limited by the extent to which they have healed themselves.

Who are you? Have you asked yourself this question? Are you willing to consider this question now or reconsider any prior answers? Let's explore it. Perhaps you will find that the quality of either answer will be deeper and more truthful after this activity.

Do the A-B-Cs and sit with this question. In your journal make a list, run with it, do not miss a label or persona that remains as an answer to who you are. Some are necessary, some you chose, and others seem to chose you. Once you have completed that, reconsider the items in the list and underline the most accurate and meaningful. Try them on, so to speak, by closing your eyes and saying each to yourself, "I am _____ ." Notice what each feels like in your body and heart. To what degree do you resonate with each? Is it truly you or a label you identify with?

Again, pare down the list by circling the ones that feel most real for you. Once again, try them on and sense their true fit. Star the one or the couple that are the closest to your innermost identity or search deeper for what answers this question.

The next question is for "each identity" to answer. Relax, don the identity and ask it these questions: "What do you want? What do you want me to know?" If tears try to surface, allow them. Any fidgeting, repositioning, yawning and changes in breathing patterns could be a wordless answers – allow, observe and go with them – to release, restore and restructure your being into healthy alignment.

Use your journal to write what you learn about who you truly are.

In *The Secret Life of Water*, Masaru Emoto imparts, "If you feel lost, disappointed, hesitant, or weak, return to yourself, to who you are, here and now and when you get there, you will discover yourself, like a lotus flower in full bloom, even in a muddy pond, beautiful and strong."[5] Consciousness dwells in you as you, as you. It is how you are deeply called to be in this world and make it your world by being you. What world do you want? What expression of yourself do you desire to bring to your family, patients, employer and into your world? No doubt, nothing less than your highest self and the highest expression of yourself. You deserve to live a high vibrational and conscious life – healthy, resilient and passionate. Expressing this in today's challenging milieu is a disruptive technology, yet a necessity. Cultivate the energy and health necessary for your well-being first, so it is a foundation for your influence, leadership and work.

Envision your high vibrational self and life from the perspective as if it is already yours. Engage all senses in this vision, feel and experience it as real now. Dwell here and let it marinate into your awareness and being. Return to this vision and state often to build the neurochemistry necessary to support and actualize the expression of your highest vibrational self and life. This yin way of being there will become your *knowing* and your *way*. Make notes in your journal affirming your feelings of aliveness including what you are grateful for *in-the-moment* of your visualization. Summarize any thing from the self inquiry above that you wish in your journal.

Zedd, a German Musician said, "Being yourself is what will make you survive through anything. If you make music to please someone, it's the first step in the wrong direction. Always do what you believe in, no matter what people say. Only way to go!"

Workplace Paradox

There are many paradoxes for a nurse, with a yin career in an environment structured by a yang model. Stress is abundant, and it is easy to succumb to the prevailing workplace model to maintain the food on your table. While this environment is risky on multiple fronts, how and where does the real you fit in? Whether subtle or blatant, hostile work environments with bullying occur between peers, ranks and disciplines among nurses and in healthcare organizations. Seniority, job stability, recognition and any withholding of it, breed competition.[6] You may also be subjected to suppression or omissive measures by co-workers or managers if you stand out or step up. How can this occur in a system claiming to care and care for health?

Gallup research on well-being found that team-level engagement was 70% impacted by the manager.[7] In a presentation by Dr. Deepak Chopra, he reveals that he assists in well-being data interpretation collected by Gallop, known for its research via polls. He explained the results show that a worker's engagement, productivity, and health are part of career and workplace wellness, and are directly influenced by their supervisor, manager or boss. The following information highlights some of the details. If a worker is ignored, their rate of disengagement goes up by 45% and they are more likely to get sick. If they are criticized, they will get better by 20-25%. So people would rather be criticized than ignored because at least they exist. Finding only one positive trait and giving an authentic recognition will decrease the worker's disengagement to less than 1%.[8] Why do managers use such tactics rather than acknowledgement when they want engagement and productivity?[9]

The current means to throttle up efficiency and productivity in business is to further mechanize work and increase use of technology over people. In a people business like healthcare, this seems counter productive. This reduces certain employment options and can disengage people due to lack of creativity, influence or ability to make a difference with their special talents.

As a human resource in a business, productivity is funded by your vital energy. You are held to some unspoken standard that you not discuss salary, fairness or work environment. Your energy is a commodity of real value, but you need enough of it for your health. Is this a paradoxical competition for your energy?

Nurses have dangerous jobs with high risk but without hazard pay, recognition or award. When injured, they are sometimes treated with malice and disregard by employers. As Terry Cawthorn, an injured-on-the-job nurse expressed, "I had poured my life into nursing. And when I got hurt, I meant nothing. I was absolutely nothing to the hospital."[10] "The Economics of Wellbeing" report states to business managers and CEOs that "The research on this topic is quite clear: Your workforce's wellbeing directly affects your organization's bottom line."[11]

Medicine is yang, reliant upon well defined boundaries and deliberate repetitive practices to address diagnosable symptoms, while attempting to provided safe predictable outcomes. Nursing is yin by its nature, with less of a container because it is practiced beyond the boundaries, often in the realm of the intangible. There is an intimacy revealed in the practice of nursing because it cultivates the heart and health of people who are unique and boundless with infinite possibility. It is paradoxical that your job, in the medical model, is mechanizing your work to a cadence of productivity. It is progressively and necessarily defining your work with deliberate repetitive practices that squeeze the space and time vitally necessary for health to be maintained for yourself and cultivated with your patients. Developing the ability to hold space for the yin and yang while creating ways for balance and health is your *response-ability* and doing so ignites your empowerment. You are the leader you seek, the cultivator of your well-being. You are the heart that rocks health care.

Tall Poppy

In her *Huffington Post* article, "Tall Poppy", Carol Vallone Mitchell, PhD, recounts the meaning of this Australian cultural phrase. What she

write, illuminates the essence of risk a tall poppy must face while realizing its full potential. She explains:

"It refers to people who stand out for their high abilities, envi-
able qualities, and/or visible success. But standing out, in this
case, isn't viewed positively. In a society that prides itself on
egalitarian principles, rising above the pack is considered anti-
social and counter cultural. Tall poppies generate hostility and
elicit a host of undermining behaviors to bring them down a
peg. This compelling desire to cut high achievers down to size is
called the 'tall poppy syndrome'."[12]

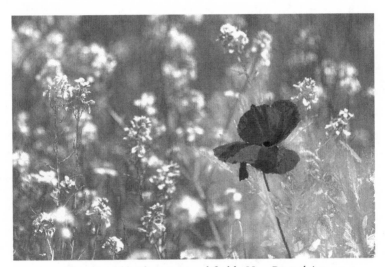

Photo in public domain - modified by Vivo Digital Arts

It is hostile for a manager to belittle, minimize, ignore or subvert
opportunity from a Tall Poppy. However, it is common to do so in a
paradigm based upon scarcity and competition. If you have a creative
or entrepreneurial spirit, you may need to find the courage to get into a
position or organization that welcomes those qualities, or leave to blaze
a new trail. Dr. Mitchell concludes her informative and motivational
article with a statement of wisdom:

"Women who lead do stand out, but the ones who are successful
are collaborative, inclusive and make themselves approachable

and relate-able. They avoid the sharp clippers that stand at the ready to cut down tall poppies."[13]

R. Buckminster Fuller, an early-to-mid-twentieth century architect, engineer, systems theorist, writer, inventor, and futurist would probably agree as he said, "You never change things by fighting the existing reality. To change things, build a new model that makes the existing model obsolete."[14] There are things that we cannot change. Then there are things that we can change that actually change things. Caring for your health is one such thing. I hope that you have gathered an evolving familiarity with your power, influence, and ability to change from this book and the heart activities included.

Transformation

Bless that which is broken, angry, painful, scary, even regretful and shameful. Where possible, learn from it. Make self-reflection a tool you skillfully use for transformation. Then *shift* your nervous system via your breath and emotions into your power of heart. Research by the HeartMath Institute has proven that heart-based thoughts, feelings and emotions affect your biology and people around you. With this, you are powerful beyond all measure if you take positive action in the direction of your heart-inspired health, dreams and purpose. Along with recognition as a nurse comes empowerment and influence, and even more profoundly when you step up and live it.

To support this from another, perhaps surprising perspective, we are amidst a transformational time. It is a time when the Western healthcare system is being called *over burdened*, *less effective* and even **broken** a time when financial and human resource energy scales need rebalancing... and a time when it may seem technology is taking over the reins. How is this transformational? Because even though science is gaining a deeper understanding of humans, humanity, health and technology, there are cracks in the methods and means that brought our health, cultures and the world to where they are now. Transformation is about rising from what is. Make achieving one's highest human potential the new frontier by pursuing just that. Self-regulation and well-being are innovative disruptive technologies to stress and illness. As a nurse, you know *things* even if your job seems to be valuing or validating them less. Reposition yourself for health. You are the conduit of care that allows any profession, hospital, business, organization or technology to touch people.

Please do not forget what you intuitively know. Instead, pause and reawaken it. You know pain and suffering and how to bridge it. You have seen resilience and amazing recovery. You know the magic of eye contact, listening, touch and connection. The reason you can give medical treatments, with a smile despite being stressed, is because you intrinsically know the magic of a warm smile and how to see beauty. Consider these benefits and blessings to those who need them.

You must accept your stress as the setup for transformation. As you do, you will increase your power and be influential. It starts with taking care of yourself and being a healthy role model, clear communicator and confident contributor of your knowledge and ideas. When you take action and *shift* to success, you become the research and the results. Teaching from knowledge is a necessary thing, but teaching from experience and leading by example is much more influential and effective. In doing so, you will need to recognize when you have the opportunity to influence and when you risk being perceived as a Tall Poppy. When you stand up and dare to make a difference because it is the right thing to do, and act from values in virtuous ways, you enlist the powerful *force of heart*.

Re-Awaken the Heart of Nursing

Now is a time for you to dig into your cobwebbed memories of why you went into nursing. You and your fellow nurses need to bring forward what you *know* about health and well-being, and about nursing. Not just the procedural skills (nursing theory, care plans, and nursing and interventions) but the people skills, health skills, life skills and skills of the heart.

Historically women entered the workforce as nurses during the wars of yesteryear. Today we have more wars going on in healthcare than ever – war on drugs, opioids, cancer and chronic disease. No wonder you have become tired and stressed.

Nurses have been on the front lines and in the trenches recognizably since the 1700s.[15] Nurses have stood by the poor, the infirm and the dying. Nurses have stood for the weak, the homeless, and the under-privileged. Nurses know of the human spirit and of the art of caring. Different from diagnosing, treating, administering medications and in-tervening in emergencies, nurses know the power of belief, presence, dignity and touch. We have much to remember, ourselves to rejuvenate and a healthy future to create, and then we must stay faithful to our purpose.

One of my professors in nursing school challenged our class, saying, "Nurses need to create our unique body of knowledge and establish ourselves as professionals to be respected. We need to maintain our au-tonomy and eventually charge for our services!" I think what my profes-sor referred to and nursing theorists have pondered is the same – health and well-being is our body of knowledge as givers of care to all, includ-ing ourselves.

How much time do you spend on the job tracking down supplies, medications or other care team members, troubleshooting computer devices, data entry, and tracking down orders or lab results? Studies mentioned in the article, "Bring Nurses Back to the Bedside," by Rhon-da Collins MSN, RN, have shown you generally spend less than two hours of a 12 hour shift on direct patient care. Yet, outcomes research shows that having you at the bedside improves outcomes and there is a positive correlation with the time you are there. This is a big motivator for hospitals in the current day of value-based purchasing, even though it is making nurses into, as some have named, data entry clerks and customer service agents rather than partners-in-care with the patient.[16]

Perhaps previously you have thought, "I'm a nurse, what more do you want me to do?" Hopefully an answer is becoming clearer to you. If you choose, your role can be the vehicle for you to be more effective. You can then start intentionally manifesting the physiology of success and health which will flow into your work and emanate to those around you.

Be willing and eager to develop a healthy *psycho-neuro-physiology* and internal environment. Your *shift* into a new frequency is an influential presence that attracts and guides others such as your family, colleagues and patients. In this way, you are like the "imaginal cells" that influence other cells to transform from the DNA expression as a caterpillar into the DNA expression of a butterfly. It is helpful to know that imaginal cells initially act separately, but then join together to create change that *shifts* them into their new order of existence. Shine your heart light on the path and walk toward your picture... then fly!

Time to Make a Difference

In 2008, The Robert Wood Johnson Foundation (RWJF) and the Institute of Medicine (IOM), founded in 1970 and renamed the National Academy of Medicine (NAM) in 2015[17], launched "a two-year initiative to respond to the need to assess and transform the nursing profession."[18] This report was to "make recommendations for an action-oriented blueprint for the future of nursing."[19] At first this made me wonder if nurses ever made recognition as professionals. This report, however, used the word "profession" when referring to nursing. In 2010, the IOM released "The Future of Nursing: Leading Change, Advancing Health." They presented that nurses should "practice to the full extent of their education and training" and in fact be "encouraged to improve via higher education." Additionally they proposed nurses to "be full partners with physicians and other health care professionals in redesigning the health care in the United States."[20] The vision from *The Future of Nursing* is continuing for the next decade via "an ad hoc committee under the auspices of the National Academies of Sciences, Engineering, and Medicine... [to] chart a path for the nursing profession to help our nation create a culture of health, reduce health disparities, and improve the health and well-being of the U.S. population in the 21st century."[21]

Though your employer may not be ready, leaders of mainstream medicine are offering both opportunities and responsibility for nurses to step up and take part in the improvement of the medical healthcare system. We are at a time when nurses are being asked to step up and teach what they know, lead, manage and innovate. Nurses are being offered power and influence. It is imperative to accept these with awareness, courage and wisdom. Nurses can evolve as the balancing principle for healthcare. The intent must not be to dominate or to act like a doctor behind nursing credentials, but to care for and teach health through maintenance and recovery.

The seed of yin (nursing) needs to grow into dynamic balance with the yang (medical model). A difficult factor is that, as a whole, nurses are at their lowest quality of personal health. It is imperative you cultivate your well-being through self-care and regulation. You also need a healthy relationship with your inner wisdom to guide your voice as you step up and influence critical decisions. You remember the Shuar Chiefs. They want you to change the dream, the paradigm and the culture. Reconnect with nature, create a well developed yin nursing model of caring for health and – as the Shuar challenged American women – get healthy. Step into your power. Be influential. Author Nora Ephron encourages, "Above all, be the heroine of your life, not the victim."

What ways have you started taking care of yourself since you began reading this book? The power of maintaining and creating health is in your hands. From this empowerment, write a slogan for your life. Be spontaneous and enthusiastic. Journal about ideas, resistance or excitement as you ponder this slogan.

Now write a slogan for the healthcare system you envision. Be creative. Let it reveal qualities of the healthcare system that you want to devote your life of work to and have take care of you and your family when needed.

Journal about ideas, resistance or excitement as you ponder this slogan.

Be a Daring Nurse Leader

I was fortunate to have a mom who shared her thoughts with me and guided me by her wisdom. Here I adapt one her pearls to apply it to nurse leadership. "Make yourself into the nurse you would want to lead, if you were the nurse manager you would want to lead you." I suggest that by applying what you learn from using the AH SUCCESS Process, you can become that leader! You do not have to be at the front of the line to lead. You can lead from the bedside, home or community, but lead you must. If the word lead is scary to you, then process that too. You may find that it is more like a movement for you, from within you, one *shift* at a time, to acknowledge and act on this calling.

This takes courage. You already act courageously in a code or when someone is overwhelmed from the impact of their diagnosis. You are no stranger to courage. Nursing offers circumstances for courage to emerge in the face of fear or resistance. But as a nurse, you are also used to the safe confines of following rules and guidelines, and gaining approval by conforming. If you truly desire to be motivated by your stress rather than devoured by it, then be willing to push your own evolution.

This means increasing your skill "to listen, learn to have tough conversations, look for joy, share pain, be more curious than defensive, be authentic rather than just fit in, all while seeking moments of togetherness."[22] Have the courage to always choose to come from compassion with yourself, your family, patients, colleagues, managers, boards and community.

The amazing thing is that now you are being asked and given permission to influence care, share your knowledge and ideas, sit in the boardroom, and teach what you know. The new Future of Nursing 2020-2030 committee at the National Academy of Medicine has charted "a path for the nursing profession to help our nation create a culture of health, reduce health disparities, and improve the health and well-being of the U.S. population."[23] This is a yang medical perspective. The strength, wisdom and yin leadership by nurses is needed to lead the direction of their health and profession. You are being called to be what Dr. Brené Brown calls a "daring leader."[24] She describes leadership as, "...

not about titles, status, and wielding power. A leader is anyone who takes responsibility for recognizing the potential in people and ideas and has the courage to develop that potential."[25]

Yes You!

Your chance of being born as who you are today was calculated by Dr. Ali Binazi to be "1 in 10 to the 2,685,000 power or a 10 followed by 2,685,000 zeroes, which is basically zero!"[26] As an author, happiness engineer and personal growth consultant, he says, "A miracle is an event so unlikely as to be almost impossible. By that definition, I've just proven that you are a miracle."[27] At the same time that you are a miracle, you are also very purposefully here, now.

Remember, Marianne Williamson's endearing and haunting question from the Preface? "Who are you not, to be?"... healthy, influential, inspirational, a leader, an agent of positive exchange or a healer.[28] You and the other heart-based nurses have the power like that of "the hand that rocks the cradle."[29] The poem refers to "motherhood as the preeminent force for change in the world."[30] You are *the heart that rocks health care*. As Marianne Williamson further insights in her poem, "Your playing small does not serve you or the world." Why? Because "...as [you] let [your] own light shine, [you] unconsciously give other people permission to do the same. As [you] are liberated from [your] own fear, [your] presence automatically liberates others."[31] The necessary *shift* is a rebalancing one, from the head to the heart. For the current healthcare system this could be a challenging distance to bridge. But if people *shift*, it's by natural order that other *shifts* will follow.

Please be generous toward yourself, give your best to your patients and lead people and your profession in the care of health. Raise up your knowledge, experience and insights and move from stress to success. Lead with your heart. Live fully as the miracle that you are. Humanity is calling. You hear it, you feel it, you know it.

(🖐) Journal about how you are feeling. What inclinations do you have for moving forward in your health, joy, life and work? Short-term pleasures and long-term goals are both important. Explore the marvel of realizing that you are a miracle. Extend that realization to everyone you meet, through you actions and intentions acknowledge they are too.

Join your colleagues who are getting healthy, lobbying, and becoming board members for organizations. Nurses are starting businesses for nursing-based child day-care, home health, long term in-home and hospice care, advocacy, and well-being consultation. What is your deepest calling? Consider that Frederick Buechner said, "Our calling is where our deep gladness and the world's hunger meet."[32]

CHAPTER 17

MOVING FORWARD

You have accomplished much by the positive action of reading this book and progressing through the empowering AH SUCCESS Process. A confused mind cannot move forward. By looking within, you have seen through your fears, doubts and perceptions to experience yourself and expand your understanding through that experience. You are probably feeling the vitality of your awakened awareness in your being, and knowledge within your mind, along with anticipatory pressure. You are feeling power as yet to-be-realized potential. Like a flower bud from a seed that once contained it all, you are destined to burst forth into full expression.

To rest on the laurels of any success is to stop growing. Growth is perpetually imminent if you are alive and stress resilient. Everything cell in your body grows and every organ renews as a result of it. New opportunity follows accomplishment because of the naturally progressive expression of life and self through creativity.

How are you feeling about your experience of stress? How are you feeling about your self and your well-being? How is that different from the feeling you had that led you to this book? What obstacles have you overcome? Which stepping stones have evolved where there once were none? What is your outlook? Make notes in your journal to answer these questions, and to highlight your shifts and accomplishments both internal and external. Also describe your new *picture*.

A Heroine's Journey

"A change of feeling is a change of destiny..." according to author Neville Goddard, "Change your conception of yourself and you will automatically change the world in which you live."[1] Maybe you were heading for ill-health and dis-empowerment. I deeply hope you feel you have *shifted*. What is next for you? The miraculous *renew-abilty* of life actually brings you not merely to the end of learning the Process or the end of this book, but to another beginning in your own growth along the road where life may push you. You may want to resist this decisive point. But you must risk revealing yourself. You are meant to overcome the ache, alchemize your new wisdom and bring it into the world for its healing. This is commonly recognized as the hero's journey.[2] However, the means by which you took this journey, the AH SUCCESS Process, was yin – inward and metaphysical – which is the way of the heroine's journey.[3] Both journey's are an adventure. The hero leaves home to return for recognition and goes back out into the world with his merits. Whereas the heroine returns home (to heart) to satisfy her quest for harmony and wholeness by balancing opposing forces such as masculine and feminine, yin and yang, life and death, and illness and health. When she accomplishes this *within*, the world *without* heals. No matter one's gender, all cycle repeatedly through both journey's.

I have walked the steps of the AH SUCCESS Process. It is how I began to heal from a work-environment burn-out. I drew upon all I knew and discovered more as I wrote the steps into this book to share this information, this wisdom, with you. With this accomplishment and a return to heart, I found myself at yet another beginning because I heard the call Guillaume Apollinaire, a French poet, wrote about:

> Come to the edge, Life said.
> They said: We are afraid.
> Come to the edge, Life said.
> They came.
> It pushed them...
> And they Flew.[4]

On the Edge

As I completed this second edition, our world was different from 2018 when I wrote the first edition of this book. Who could have known in the year for which the chant was "2020 Vision", *Life* would push people's immune systems and healthcare workers so hard. Nurses, already fatigued and stressed from the prodromal crises in healthcare, were blind-sided by extremely hazardous work conditions. You faced frustrating limits of medical scope, knowledge and treatments, the finite availability of staff, supplies, equipment and resources, and limitations of time, energy, influence and life. The worldwide medical disaster required untold amounts of stamina, and you and your colleagues were left with your ingenuity and heart to get through, often behind a wall at an intravenous line's length from your isolated, lonely, scared, suffering often sedated patients. This was a moral injury for you personally as the most trusted professional. The only cure for this deep harm is forgiveness, starting with yourself.

You are a heroine of stellar magnitude with the heart of a healer. Feel gracious for your fortitude and your amazing, responsive and commanding sympathetic nervous system that sustained you. If it wasn't sputtering before, it likely is now. You may feel depleted, as if your soul has receded behind a vacant stare of fatigue. Breathe a fresh air filled breath for yourself. You are a survivor; you are alive.

The cumulative effects of emotional trauma and powerlessness can heal in parasympathetic dominant neuro-bio-chemistry and fellowship. Teach and learn with your colleagues how to *co-create* health. The A-B-Cs will soothe and the AH SUCCESS Process is a helpful guide for you to act in your best interest. As needed, follow your heart and be drawn to practitioners who will facilitate repletion of your stress-ravaged body and rejuvenation of your well-being. It is a pilgrimage back to health, a heroine's journey. You are integral to the empathetic, wisdom-based future of caring for health.

Miracles Happen

In each moment of each day you have a choice of what you will let into your mind, body and life. You choose what you will let go and what you will create. Will you manifest love or fear, peace or war, parasympathetic or sympathetic effects, well-being or dis-ease?

Inspirational wisdom says, "There are only two ways to live your life. One is as though nothing is a miracle. The other is as though everything is a miracle."[6] Each breath-cycle completes a moment and delivers you to the beginning of the miraculous next. Because you are alive, you can *shift* your perception to create health and vitality in your body, your relationships, your job, and in your little corner of the world. Like the heroine's transformation, this *'shift in perception'* – from fear to love, limit to limitless, separate to wholeness, lack to abundance, from stress to success – is the miracle, according to A Course in Miracles, and "only miracles can be the result from doing so."[7]

You Are A Miracle

As a nurse, you are *the heart that rocks health care.* You are a *heroine.* The work you do is miraculous – warming possibilities, rekindling healing glows, resuscitating lives and touching souls. You possess power to heal and to influence healing, which is miraculous. When you do the steps to **center** and **elevate**, you will become empowered as a healthier and more influential force for your self and others. You will ask deeper and clearer questions, and see more options and solutions in a more holistic way that embraces the tenets of Yin-Yang. The world needs your best expression of yourself.

A New Paradigm

The secret is You, the nurse, are the *Spirit* of any organization or system. Without you it is just a shell of rules, agendas, files and processes, a concept. The system depends upon you to exist, *co-operate.* Caring is your way as a nurse. Your work is doing that which you are here to do in the *way of your heart*. You are empowered and influential by way of your knowledge and from opening yourself to the personal experience of others. You know about regulating your response by feeling beyond and thinking above your immediate experience and physiology. You have skills that cultivate and build capacity for compassion, creativity, cognition, communication, performance and, yes, to co-create health. With your inner wisdom, nursing and medical knowledge, you walk between worlds and remain influential because you can communicate in the respective language of each.

Now is the time for the balance of dualities into wholeness and to find your way forward.

Your role is crucial at a time when happiness, which correlates with well-being and illness, is on the decline (even prior to 2020) in the most technologically developed countries – none ranking in the top ten, including the U.S.[8,9] Concurrently, recent estimates suggest that "one third to one half of all jobs could be replaced by artificial intelligence in the next two decades".[10] This seems to have been exasperated by the global health crisis of 2020. The full expression of the strength of your role as a nurse and presence as Soul will bring holistic principles and wholeness into the system's paradigm. You can integrate information from multiple paradigms to envision a new, holistic way that maximizes caring for health as a way of life and as needed, incorporate the safe use of technology and medical interventions.

This is an opportune moment in time for each of us play an integral role the many burdened medical systems of the West. David Grubin's film, "RX: The Quiet Revolution", speaks to it clearly. The Western system of healthcare needs a new model because "A disease-based, doctor-centered medicine served us well for the first half of the 20th century, but economic pressures and a changing population are revealing its shortcomings."[11]

The *busy-ness* of doing the tasks and services of a job can deprive *caring* when exchanged for efficiency, competition and productivity. For the sake of your well-being and that of your family and patients, let nothing separate your heart from what you do or how you do it, including caring for yourself – not a job, relationship or the headlines.

This separation is what I see as deeply foundational to the experience of stress in nurses and the creation of chronic ill-health in our culture as a casualty of the Western Healthcare model.

The sea of stress, fear and illness can be wide and challenging to navigate. But you must navigate it for yourself and those in your care despite any chaos or distractions you may encounter. The journey leads you back to yourself, to your 'hearth' which is the wholeness and holiness of heart, home and health.

Your Success

As you *move forward,* use the AH SUCCESS process and its principles often and as you see fit. Be increasingly *aware. Shift* your state of consciousness to one that supports vitality. Be *open to the possible.* Seek experiences of *awe* and *wonder.* Live in coherence and from your *heart* because the ancient Essene texts reveal, with coherence "mountains will move."[12] Your coherence of thought, feeling, emotion, nervous system and heart will affect your health and world, and will align those around you.

As Caroline Myss, five-time New York Times bestselling author and internationally renowned speaker in the fields of human consciousness, spirituality and mysticism, health, energy medicine, and the science of medical intuition says, "All life breathes together."

Inspire and encourage your sister and brother colleagues, and *co-create* a community of nurses healing hearts and living naturally healthy lives on a healthy planet. Model and teach health to others through your chosen career, vocation, business or way of being. Help unburden the future of healthcare by leading a *shift* to a hearty, healthy paradigm.

One More Thing

Thank you for taking time for yourself and sharing that time with me via this book. I hope that it has *re-awakened* great reverence toward your work and facilitated awakening to the evolution ahead as individuals, nurses, and as a global community. Be a model for and encourage every individual to aspire to cultivate peace and health within themselves.

In Chapter 5, I shared my personal introduction to the concept and beginning of my contemplation of the question, "How is a healing of one being a healing of all beings?" After years of awareness, learning and practicing, I had an inspiration. It arose poetically while creating an integrative healing arts class for nurses. I hope that the resulting poem shared below sheds some light for you.

What Do I See?

What do I see, Patient,
what do I see?
When I look at you,
could you be me?

You appear there,
as far as I see.
Through knowing you,
could I better know me?

What's that feeling inside me...
when you're in pain,
I want to relieve?
When you feel alone,
with you I'm drawn to be?

There's a whisper, a tug,
a knowing, you see.
Despite the numbers and graphs
all looking perfectly.

There is something I know differently.
Some kind of Inner technology.

Somehow we're connected,
breath... mind... whatever it be.
It is an illusion
that we live separately.

The circle of life,
ebb and flow of energy.
A dance of the cosmos
that happens in 'We'.

Two sides of the same,
brought together are we.
Where calling meets need,
there is purpose, you see.

So that part in you
is honored by that part in me –
Eternal and loving,
that will never cease to be.

Can you see, Patient,
that which I see?
As we both struggle
with time, illness and money?

We will bless these things
and let them be.
We must meet beyond –
where you are me.

— *Barbara Young RN, 2017*

The secret to moving from stress to success is to *live with heart*. Wholeness comes by way of the heart because it connects all as one.

Real-ization of this is transformational. You *are* the *Heart that Rocks Health Care.*

Come to the edge.

Dare to lead.

Let the healing of all beings start with your healing.

To your heart-inspired success!

Barbara

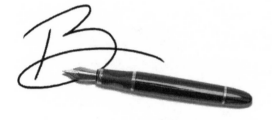

SUPPORTING MATERIALS
ⓘ

Additional materials and further reading
recommendations are available at:

https://BYoungBooks.com/support-heart

PROFESSIONAL RESOURCES

American Holistic Nurses Association
   https://www.ahna.org/

American Holistic Nurses Credentialing Corporation
   http://www.ahncc.org/

Campaign for Action
   https://campaignforaction.org/

The Institute for Functional Medicine
   https://www.ifm.org

Institute of Medicine / National Academy of Medicine

Healthy Nurse, Healthy Nation – ANA Enterprise

Robert Wood Johnson Foundation
   https://www.rwjf.org/

Note: Author has or has had no financial or other beneficial
   interest with any of the above resources except
   BYoungBooks.com. She is a member of AHNA and
   credentialed via AHNCC.

ENDNOTES

"Give credit where credit is due,"

— Origin unclear, sources suggest Samuel Adams

Endnotes - Preface

1   Rose. 2013. "What Do Nurses Want from Their Leaders?" Emerging Nurse Leader. May 23, 2013. https://www.emergingrnleader.com/ emerging-nurse-leadership/

2   Maxwell, John C. 2008. The 21 Irrefutable Laws of Leadership. Nashville, TN: Thomas Nelson

3   Brown Brene. 2019. Dare to Lead: Brave Work, Tough Conversations, Whole Hearts. New York: Random House

4   Marianne Williamson, "Our Deepest Fear" (poem), A Return to Love: Reflections on the Principles of A Course in Miracles, Harper Perennial, 2012, ©1992

Endnotes - Chapter 1

1   "America's #1 Health Problem," The American Institute of Stress (blog), Accessed December 29, 2018, https://www.stress.org/americas-1-health-problem

2   "What Is Functional Medicine? | IFM." The Institute for Functional Medicine, www.ifm.org/functional-medicine/what-is-functional-medicine/

3   Soleil, Gina. "Workplace Stress: The Health Epidemic of the 21st Century." HuffPost, HuffPost, 7 Dec. 2017, www.huffpost.com/entry/ workplace-stress-the-heal_b_8923678.

4   "What Is Functional Medicine? | IFM." The Institute for Functional Medicine, www.ifm.org/functional-medicine/what-is-functional-medicine/
Functional Medicine is a systems biology–based approach that focuses on identifying and addressing the root cause of disease. Each symptom or differential diagnosis may be one of many contributing to an individual's illness. A diagnosis can be the result of more than one cause. For example, depression can be caused by many different factors, including inflammation. Likewise, a cause such as inflammation may lead to a number of different diagnoses, including depression. The precise manifestation of each cause depends on the individual's genes, environment and lifestyle, and only treatments that address the right cause will have lasting benefit beyond symptom suppression.

5   H. J. Eysenck (1990), "Type A Behavior and Coronary Heart Disease: The Third Stage", Journal of Social Behavior and Personality, 5: 25–44

6   Author's Note: Self-regulation basically involves controlling one's behavior, emotions, impulses and thoughts such as thinking before you act and the ability to pick yourself up after a disappointment. On a deeper and more profound level, it involves the ability to act consistent with your deepest values and by using

instinctual and innate bodily functions, to regulate the body by profoundly and effectively shifting its physiology to positively affect stress, health, relationships, success and influence.

7 Michael Garko, PhD, "The Terrain Within: A Naturalistic Way to Think," Lets Talk Nutrition, Accessed July 05, 2019. http://letstalknutrition.com/the-terrain-within-a-naturalistic-way-to-think/
Louis Pasteur (1822-1895) is purported to have made this statement on his deathbed. The origin of the quote is attributed to Claude Bernard (1813-1878), a physiologist and contemporary of Pasteur. By quoting Bernard, Pasteur was recanting his germ theory, a theory that assigned the cause of disease to microbes invading and reeking havoc on the body, with specific germs causing specific diseases.

8 Ralph Metzner, 2014, "The Causes of Disease: The Great Debate." Functional Medicine University - The Leader in Online Training in Functional Diagnostic Medicine, July 17, 2014, https://www.functionalmedicineuniversity.com/public/937.cfm

9 "Environment," Dictionary.com, Dictionary.com, Accessed May 6, 2019, https://www.dictionary.com/browse/environment?s=t

10 David Rettew, 2017, "Nature Versus Nurture: Where We Are in 2017, Psychology Today, Sussex Publishers, October 6, 2017, https://www.psychologytoday.com/us/blog/abcs-child-psychiatry/201710/nature-versus-nurture-where-we-are-in-2017
The questions involves whether human behavior is driven by innate biological forces or the product of our learning and environment.

Endnotes - Chapter 2

1 Harvard Health Publishing. "Understanding the Stress Response." Harvard Health, www.health.harvard.edu/staying-healthy/understanding-the-stress-response
Excellent overview of 'fight-or-flight' and the stress response. It further explains how frequent and chronic activation of this survival mechanism via the sympathetic nervous system keeps the body on high alert and impairs health.

2 "Classical Conditioning," Wikipedia, Wikimedia Foundation, 24 Aug. 2018, en.wikipedia.org/wiki/Classical conditioning
Classical conditioning (also known as Pavlovian or respondent conditioning) refers to a learning procedure in which a biologically potent stimulus (e.g. food) is paired with a previously neutral stimulus (e.g. a bell). It also refers to the learning process that results from this pairing, through which the neutral stimulus comes to elicit a response (e.g. salivation) that is usually similar to the one elicited by the potent stimulus. These basic facts, which require many qualifications, were first studied in detail by Ivan Pavlov through experiments with dogs.

3 Alexandra Robbins, 2015, "The Problem With Satisfied Patients," The Atlantic. Atlantic Media Company, April 17, 2015, https://www.theatlantic.com/health/archive/2015/04/the-problem-with-satisfied-patients/390684/

4 Blegen, Mary A, et al. "Baccalaureate Education in Nursing and Patient Outcomes." The Journal of Nursing Administration, U.S. National Library of Medicine, Feb. 2013, www.ncbi.nlm.nih.gov/pubmed/23314788

5 ibid

6 ibid

7   "Nursing Quality Greatly Influences Patient Outcomes | PNW." Purdue
    Northwest Online, 11 Sept. 2017, nursingonline.pnw.edu/articles/nursing-
    quality-influences-patient-outcomes.aspx

8   "The Future of Nursing: Leading Change, Advancing Health." The Future
    of Nursing: Leading Change, Advancing Health, 19 Oct. 2018, www.
    nationalacademies.org/hmd/Reports/2010/The-Future-of-Nursing-Leading-
    Change-Advancing-Health.aspx

9   "Robert Wood Johnson Foundation Launches Initiative to Support Academic
    Progression in Nursing." RWJF, 21 July 2015, www.rwjf.org/en/library/articles-
    and-news/2012/03/robert-wood-johnson-foundation-launches-initiative-to-
    support-ac.html

10 "About Chronic Disease," n.d., Rep. About Chronic Disease, Washington, DC:
    National Health Council, Found at https://www.nationalhealthcouncil.org/sites/
    default/files/AboutChronicDisease.pdf

11 "Overview - Preventing Chronic Diseases: a Vital Investment," 2015, World
    Health Organization, World Health Organization, December 21, 2015, https://
    www.who.int/chp/chronic_disease_report/part1/en/index1.html

12 "Chronic Diseases in America," n.d., Centers for Disease Control and Prevention,
    Centers for Disease Control and Prevention, Accessed July 28, 2019, https://www.
    cdc.gov/chronicdisease/resources/infographic/chronic-diseases.htm

13 "Almanac of Chronic Disease 2009," 2009, Rep, Almanac of Chronic Disease
    2009, Parership to Fight Chronic Disease, Access online at http://www.
    fightchronicdisease.org/sites/default/files/docs/2009AlmanacofChronicDisea
    se_updated81009.pdf

14 Haddad, Lisa M. "Nursing Shortage." StatPearls [Internet]., U.S. National Library
    of Medicine, 19 Jan. 2019, www.ncbi.nlm.nih.gov/books/NBK493175/

15 "Registered Nurses : Occupational Outlook Handbook." 2019. U.S. Bureau of
    Labor Statistics. U.S. Bureau of Labor Statistics. September 4, 2019. https://www.
    bls.gov/ooh/healthcare/registered-nurses.htm

16 Jennifer Gerson Uffalussy, "Nurses Are Some of the Unhealthiest Americans and
    We Need to Help Change That", Yahoo! News, Yahoo!, 6 May 2017, www.yahoo.
    com/lifestyle/nurses-unhealthiest-americans-need-help-change-150335598.html

17 ibid

18 "Burnout," n.d., Merriam-Webster, Merriam-Webster, Accessed July 28, 2019,
    https://www.merriam-webster.com/dictionary/burnout
    "burnout (noun) 1 : the cessation of operation usually of a jet or rocket engine
    also : the point at which burnout occurs 2 a : exhaustion of physical or emotional
    strength or motivation usually as a result of prolonged stress or frustration b :
    a person suffering from burnout 3 : a person showing the effects of drug abuse
    burn out (verb) 1 : to drive out or destroy the property of by fire 2 : to cause to
    fail, wear out, or become exhausted especially from overwork or overuse burn out
    (transitive verb) : to suffer burnout Antonyms: Noun refreshment, rejuvenation,
    rejuvenescence, revitalization"

19 Stimpfel, Amy Witkoski, et al. "The Longer The Shifts For Hospital Nurses,
    The Higher The Levels Of Burnout And Patient Dissatisfaction." Health Affairs
    (Project Hope), U.S. National Library of Medicine, Nov. 2012, www.ncbi.nlm.
    nih.gov/pmc/articles/PMC3608421/

20 Gouin, Jean-Philippe, and Janice K Kiecolt-Glaser. "The Impact of Psychological

Stress on Wound Healing: Methods and Mechanisms." Immunology and Allergy Clinics of North America, U.S. National Library of Medicine, Feb. 2011, www.ncbi.nlm.nih.gov/pmc/articles/PMC3052954/

21 ibid

22 Peggy Martin, 1987, Chapter 6 "The Therapeutic Use of Self," Psychiatric Nursing, SpringerLink, Palgrave, London, January 1, 1987, https://link.springer.com/chapter/10.1007/978-1-349-09408-0_6 "The therapeutic use of self is the central focus of nursing and requires that the nurse is aware of his or her own thoughts, feelings and actions."

23 Richard L. Pullen, 2010, "Fostering Therapeutic Nurse-Patient Relationships : Nursing Made Incredibly Easy," LWW, May 2010, https://journals.lww.com/nursingmadeincrediblyeasy/Fulltext/2010/05000/Fostering_therapeutic_nurse_patient_relationships.1.aspx#JCL0-1 "A therapeutic nurse-patient relationship is defined as a helping relationship that's based on mutual trust and respect, the nurturing of faith and hope, being sensitive to self and others, and assisting with the gratification of your patient's physical, emotional, and spiritual needs through your knowledge and skill."

24 "Active Listening Matters in Health Care," 2019, Concorde Career College, July 12, 2019, https://www.concorde.edu/blog/career-tips-advice/active-listening "...a Conflict Research Consortium at the University of Colorado defined active listening as "a way of listening and responding to another person that improves mutual understanding."

25 Edward M. Pallette, 2001, Nurses Know: What Happened to Health Care?: What Can We Do about It, Fullerton, CA: Empathy Pub., LLC, 296

26 Michael Edison Hayden, "Nurse Arrested for Refusing to Draw Blood from Unconscious Patient Praised for 'Heroic Act'", ABC News, ABC News Network, 2 Sept. 2017, abcnews.go.com/US/nurse-arrested-refusing-draw-blood-unconscious-patient-praised/story?id=49583337

27 Traynor, Michael. 2017. Critical Resilience for Nurses: an Evidence-Based Guide to Survival and Change in the Modern NHS. Abingdon, Oxon: Routledge is an imprint of the Taylor & Francis Group p 115

28 Jackson, Debra, Angela Firtko, and Michel Edenborough. 2007. "Personal Resilience as a Strategy for Surviving and Thriving in the Face of Workplace Adversity: a Literature Review." Journal of Advanced Nursing 60(1), 1–9 doi: 10.1111/j.1365-2648.2007.04412.x

29 "Stereotypes, Bias, Prejudice, and Discrimination, Oh My!" 2016. Psych Learning Curve. October 11, 2016. http://psychlearningcurve.org/stereotypes-bias-prejudice-and-discrimination/

30 "Gender Stereotyping." n.d. OHCHR. United Nations. Accessed July 30, 2019. https://www.ohchr.org/EN/Issues/Women/WRGS/Pages/GenderStereotypes.aspx

31 Sally Helgesen and Julie Johnson, 2010, The Female Vision: Women's Real Power at Work, San Francisco: Berrett-Koehler Publishers Inc.

32 Tyana Daley, 2016, "Why Men Should Consider Joining the Nursing Field," Minority Nurse, January 12, 2016, https://minoritynurse.com/why-men-should-consider-joining-the-nursing-field/

33 "The Coalition for Better Understanding of Nursing." 2019, YouTube, The Coalition for Better Understanding of Nursing, March 7, 2019, https://youtu.be/

qECA2-o7VJQ

34 Pavithra Mohan, 2019, "'I've Been a Nurse for 20 Years, The Male Nurses I Work with Have a Different Pay Track,'" Fast Company, Fast Company, April 4, 2019, https://www.fastcompany.com/90324489/ive-been-a-nurse-for-20-years-the-male-nurses-i-work-with-have-a-different-pay-track

35 Ulrike Muench, 2015, "Salary Differences Between US Male and Female RNs," JAMA, American Medical Association, March 24, 2015, https://jamanetwork.com/journals/jama/fullarticle/2208795#jld150006r4

36 "Debunking Nursing Stereotypes," 2017, Daily Nurse, February 6, 2017, https://dailynurse.com/debunking-nursing-stereotypes/

37 "Sunlight - White or Coloured: Spectrum, Dispersion, Videos and Examples," 2018, Toppr, April 17, 2018, https://www.toppr.com/guides/science/light/sunlight-white-or-coloured/

38 Institute of Medicine (US) Committee on the Robert Wood Johnson Foundation Initiative on the Future of Nursing, and at the Institute of Medicine, 1970, "Transforming Leadership," The Future of Nursing: Leading Change, Advancing Health, U.S. National Library of Medicine, January 1, 1970. https://www.ncbi.nlm.nih.gov/books/NBK209867/

39 Brie Isom, WSBT 22 Reporter. "How Doctors Diagnose and Treat 'burnout'." WSBT. May 30, 2019. Accessed June 1, 2019. https://wsbt.com/news/local/how-doctors-treat-burnout

40 World Health Organization. Accessed May 16, 2019. https://icd.who.int/browse11/l-m/en#/http://id.who.int/icd/entity/129180281

41 Coles, Tad B. 2017. "Compassion Fatigue and Burnout: History, Definitions and Assessment." Veterinarian's Money Digest. October 27, 2017. https://www.vmdtoday.com/journals/vmd/2017/october2017/compassion-fatigue-and-burnout-history-definitions-and-assessment
German-born American psychologist Herbert J. Freudenberger first used this term in 1974 to describe symptoms he himself had experienced: "exhaustion, disillusionment and withdrawal resulting from intense devotion to a cause that failed to produce the expected result."

42 "Burnout." n.d. Psychology Today. Sussex Publishers. Accessed July 28, 2019. https://www.psychologytoday.com/us/basics/burnout
Burnout – a state of emotional, mental, and often physical exhaustion brought on by prolonged or repeated stress – is not simply a result of working long hours.

43 Coles, op. cit.

44 Swamy, Lakshmana, David Mohr, Amanda Blok, Ekaterina Anderson, Martin Charns, Renda Soylemez Wiener, and Seppo Rinne, "Impact of Workplace Climate on Burnout Among Critical Care Nurses in the Veterans Health Administration," American Journal of Critical Care 29, no. 5 (2020): 380-89, doi:10.4037/ajcc2020831

45 David C. Holzman, 2010, "What's in a Color? The Unique Human Health Effect of Blue Light," Environmental Health Perspectives, National Institute of Environmental Health Sciences, January 2010; 118(1): A22–A27, https://www.ncbi.nlm.nih.gov/pmc/articles/PMC2831986

46 ibid

47 Kutney-Lee, Ann, et al. "Nursing: A Key To Patient Satisfaction." Health Affairs, vol. 28, no. Supplement 3, 2009, doi:10.1377/hlthaff.28.4.w669

Endnotes - Chapter 3

1   Paramahansa Yogananda, "This World Is Not the Same to All People. Each One Lives in... at QuoteTab," QuoteTab, Accessed September 12, 2019, https://www.quotetab.com/quote/by-paramahansa-yogananda/this-world-is-not-the-same-to-all-people-each-one-lives-in-his-little-domain#56eQYBWob2cIW0CI.99

2   Chevalier, Sinatra, Stephen T., Oschman, James L., Sokal, Karol, Sokal, and Pawel, 2012, "Earthing: Health Implications of Reconnecting the Human Body to the Earth's Surface Electrons," Journal of Environmental and Public Health, Hindawi, January 12, 2012, https://www.hindawi.com/journals/jeph/2012/291541/

3   ibid

4   John Perkins, "Dream Change Staff & Board," Dream Change, Accessed July 2018, www.dreamchange.org/staff-board/

5   Michael Devitt, 2018, "CDC Data Show U.S. Life Expectancy Continues to Decline." AAFP, December 10, 2018, https://www.aafp.org/news/health-of-the-public/20181210lifeexpectdrop.html

6   Rhonda Byrne, 2006, The Secret, NY, NY: Atria Publishing Group, https://amzn.to/2SR7Xsy

7   "Missing Links with Gregg Braden," Season 3 Episode 4, 2019, Missing Links, Gaia, https://www.gaia.com/lp/missing-links

8   Paul Levy, "Quantum Meta-Physics," Awaken in the Dream, 15 Feb. 2016, www.awakeninthedream.com/articles/quantum-meta-physics

9   Harvard Health Publishing, "The Power of the Placebo Effect," Harvard Health, Harvard Health Publishing (Harvard Medical School), May 2017, https://www.health.harvard.edu/mental-health/the-power-of-the-placebo-effect

10 Joe Dispenza, "How I Healed Myself After Breaking 6 Vertebrae," The Placebo Effect - How I Healed Myself After Breaking 6 Vertebrae, Dr. Joe Dispenza, www.healyourlife.com/how-i-healed-myself-after-breaking-6-vertebrae

11 "Lissa Rankin, MD - Is There Scientific Proof We Can Heal Ourselves?," 2012, TEDxAmericanRiviera, August 15, 2012, https://tedxamericanriviera.com/lissa-rankin-md-is-there-scientific-proof-we-can-heal-ourselves/

12 Alexandra Robbins, 2016, The Nurses: a Year of Secrets, Drama, and Miracles with the Heroes of the Hospital, New York: Workman

13 Olson, Ann. 2013. "The Theory of Self-Actualization." Psychology Today. Sussex Publishers. August 13, 2013. https://www.psychologytoday.com/us/blog/theory-and-psychopathology/201308/the-theory-self-actualization

14 projects, Contributors to Wikimedia. 2018. "American Writer and Lecturer." Wikiquote. Wikimedia Foundation, Inc. August 24, 2018. https://en.wikiquote.org/wiki/Dale_Carnegie
    projects, Contributors to Wikimedia. 2018. "American Author." Wikiquote. Wikimedia Foundation, Inc. January 15, 2018. https://en.wikiquote.org/wiki/Napoleon_Hill.
    projects, Contributors to Wikimedia. 2019. "Austrian Neurologist and Psychiatrist." Wikiquote. Wikimedia Foundation, Inc. October 4, 2019. https://en.wikiquote.org/wiki/Viktor_Frankl

projects, Contributors to Wikimedia. 2019. "Philosopher from Ancient Greece (C.55 - 0135)." Wikiquote. Wikimedia Foundation, Inc. September 21, 2019. https://en.wikiquote.org/wiki/Epictetus
projects, Contributors to Wikimedia. 2019. "German-Born Physicist and Founder of the Theory of Relativity." Wikiquote. Wikimedia Foundation, Inc. October 3, 2019. https://en.wikiquote.org/wiki/Albert_Einstein

15 Keller, James. n.d. "James Keller Quotes." BrainyQuote. Xplore. Accessed August 5, 2019. https://www.brainyquote.com/quotes/james_keller_192856

16 Masaru Emoto, 2004, The Hidden Messages in Water, Hillsboro, OR, Beyond Words

17 Culpepper, Jetta Carol. "Alchemy, Definition of." Merriam-Webster Online: The Language Center. 4, no. 1/2 (2000): 9-11. Accessed September 13, 2020. doi:10.1108/err.2000.4.1_2.9.11.
Alchemy: 2. a power or process that changes or transforms something in a mysterious or impressive way

18 Yin and Yang," Wikipedia, Wikimedia Foundation, 13 May 2018, en.wikipedia.org/wiki/Yin and_yang
Yin is characterized as slow, soft, yielding, diffuse, cold, wet, and passive; and is associated with water, earth, the moon, femininity, and night time. Yang, by contrast, is fast, hard, solid, focused, hot, dry, and active; and is associated with fire, sky, the sun, masculinity and daytime.

19 "Table 1.1: Current Estimates and Future Trends in Chronic Health Conditions That Interact with the Health Risks Associated with Climate Change: Climate and Health Assessment," n.d., Climate and Health Assessment, U.S. Global Change Research Program, Accessed July 24, 2018, https://health2016.globalchange.gov/climate-change-and-human-health/tables/current-estimates-and-future-trends-chronic-health-conditions

20 Shirie Leng, 2013, "The Medical Model versus the Nursing Model: A Difference in Philosophy." KevinMD.com (blog), KevinMD.com, May 13, 2013, https://www.kevinmd.com/blog/2013/05/medical-model-nursing-model-difference-philosophy.html

21 Carrie Wiita, 2018, "What Is the Medical Model? And Why Do People Seem to Hate It so Much?" By Happenchance: The Journey of a Therapist-in-Training, By Happenchance Inc., August 18, 2018, https://www.byhappenchance.com/blogroll/what-is-the-medical-model

22 Regine Birute. 2011, "The Importance of Care in Business," HuffPost, HuffPost, May 25, 2011, https://www.huffpost.com/entry/carenect_b_799793

23 "Technology," 2019, Wikipedia. Wikimedia Foundation. June 25, 2019. https://en.wikipedia.org/wiki/Technology
Technology is a "science of craft", from the Greek roots of techne meaning "art, skill, cunning of hand" and -logia meaning the collection of techniques, skills, methods, and processes... [It is used here to refer to the art and skill of care including self care and concern for others, as a human technology].

24 Joy Yang, "The Human Microbiome Project: Extending the Definition of What Constitutes a Human," National Human Genome Research Institute (NHGRI), NIH, 1 July 2012, www.genome.gov/27549400/the-human-microbiome-project-extending-the-definition-of-what-constitutes-a-human/

25 Lu Qi, 2017, "Ask the Expert: Sugary Drinks and Genetic Risk for Obesity," The Nutrition Source, November 20, 2017,

https://www.hsph.harvard.edu/nutritionsource/2012/11/19/
ask-the-expert-sugary-drinks-and-genetic-risk-for-obesity/

26 Lipton, Bruce. "Bruce Lipton, PhD." BiontologyArizona, www.biontologyarizona.
com/dr-bruce-lipton/

Endnotes - Chapter 4

1   Author's note: In the 1990's I heard this anecdote with Confucius as the one
imparting the wisdom. A current internet search attributes it to the Dalai Lama.
No definitive reference was found as to the source of the anecdote, however.
Included here with gratitude to whomever is the source, and whomever wisely
spoke the words; the message is very clear.

2   "Albrecht's Four Types of Stress: Managing Common Pressures." From MindTools.
com, Accessed August 2, 2019, www.mindtools.com/pages/article/albrecht-stress.
htm

3   "State of Patient Care in Massachusetts' Survey Released for National Nurses
Week Finds Nurses Sounding the Alarm Over Deteriorating Conditions for
Hospitalized Patients and Need for Safe Patient Limits," 2018, News & Events
- Massachusetts Nurses Association, Massachusetts Nurses Association, May 7,
2018, https://www.massnurses.org/news-and-events/p/openItem/10940

4   Rebecca Hendren, 2010, "Ten Ways to Increase Nurses' Time at the Bedside,"
HealthLeaders Media, March 16, 2010, https://www.healthleadersmedia.com/
nursing/ten-ways-increase-nurses-time-bedside

5   "To Multitask or Not to Multitask," 2018, USC Masters of Applied Psychology
Program Online, University of Southern California, July 17, 2018, https://
appliedpsychologydegree.usc.edu/blog/to-multitask-or-not-to-multitask/

6   Stacy Lu, "How Chronic Stress Is Harming Our DNA," Monitor on Psychology,
45,9, American Psychological Association, October 2014, 28, Accessed June 29,
2019, https://www.apa.org/monitor/2014/10/chronic-stress

7   Tom Beckman, "Citations for "60-90% of All Doctor's Office Visits
Are for Stress-related Ailments and Complaints," LinkedIn (blog), April
6, 2016, Accessed June 29, 2019, https://www.linkedin.com/pulse/
citations-90-all-doctors-office-visits-stress-related-tom-beckman

8   "How Stress Affects Your Body and Behavior," Mayo Clinic (blog), April 04,
2019, Accessed June 29, 2019, https://www.mayoclinic.org/healthy-lifestyle/
stress-management/in-depth/stress-symptoms/art-20050987

9   "Fact Sheet: Health Disparities and Stress," American Psychological Association,
Accessed June 29, 2019, https://www.apa.org/topics/health-disparities/
fact-sheet-stress

10 Stephen Sinatra, "Cardiologist Dr. Sinatra Explains How to Reduce Inflammation
In the Body," Dr. Sinatra's HeartMD Institute (blog), September 05, 2018,
Accessed October 29, 2019, https://heartmdinstitute.com/heart-health/
inflammation-and-disease/

11 Suzanne C. Segerstrom, and Gregory E. Miller, "Psychological Stress and
the Human Immune System: A Meta-analytic Study of 30 Years of Inquiry,"
Psychological Bulletin, July 2004, Accessed June 6, 2018, https://www.ncbi.nlm.
nih.gov/pmc/articles/PMC1361287/

12 Mohd Razali Salleh, "Life Event, Stress and Illness," The Malaysian Journal of Medical Sciences: MJMS, October 2008, Accessed October 19, 2019. https://www.ncbi.nlm.nih.gov/pmc/articles/PMC3341916/

13 https://www.aarda.org/news-information/statistics/

14 Charles W. Schmidt, "Questions Persist: Environmental Factors in Autoimmune Disease." Environmental Health Perspectives, June 2011, Accessed November 29, 2018 https://www.ncbi.nlm.nih.gov/pmc/articles/PMC3114837/

15 ibid

16 Author's note: As a per diem nurse, I carried my own PPO medical insurance that allowed me to self-refer, unlike the HMO insurance that a require a referral for specialists from a primary care doctor.

17 "Two Kinds of Physicians" - Health Professions and Prelaw Center - Indiana University Bloomington- University Division, Accessed Dec 12, 2017, www.hpplc.indiana.edu/medicine/med-res-twokinds.shtml
Two Kinds of Physicians: Allopathic and Osteopathic. There are two kinds of practicing physicians in the United States: allopathic physicians (MD's) and osteopathic physicians (DO's). Both are fully licensed physicians, trained in diagnosing and treating illnesses and disorders .and performing surgery... and in providing preventive care. However, osteopathic physicians are trained in some special areas in which allopathic physicians do not receive training.

18 Author's note: Wholistic vs Holistic - I have seen the definition of these terms change over decades and between disciplines. I understand Wholistic to suggest a well-rounded spectrum of things, options, and disciplines meaning the whole known view. I more often use the word Holistic referring to wholeness of a prismatic or holographic scope which further includes all interrelated dimensions including what appears known and unknown, seen and unseen, such as The Divine. As a holistic nurse, the latter resonates for me.

19 "What Is a Naturopathic Doctor?" Association of Accredited Naturopathic Medical Colleges (AANMC), Accessed April 17, 2018, https://aanmc.org/what-is-a-naturopathic-doctor/
NDs provide primary patient care that blends natural medicine with conventional diagnosis and treatment. Naturopathic physicians treat the cause of illness, work to prevent disease whenever possible and teach patients how to live healthy lives. NDs have many tools to treat patients, including nutrition, lifestyle medicine, physical medicine and herbal therapies.

20 Author's note: Wholistic vs Holistic - I have seen the definition of these terms change over decades and between disciplines. I understand Wholistic to suggest a well-rounded spectrum of things, options, and disciplines meaning the whole known view. I more often use the word Holistic referring to wholeness of a prismatic or holographic scope which further includes all interrelated dimensions including what appears known and unknown, seen and unseen, such as The Divine. As a holistic nurse, the latter resonates for me.

21 Author's note: Conscious Living Education™ -a holistic program I developed for self-care, lifestyle modification and mind-body skills. It was the foundation of teaching and working with my clients as a private practice Holistic Nurse Consultant. It's framework (Identification-Exploration-Application-Integration) was inspired by the concepts of the American Nurses Association's Nursing Process which I was trained to use in nursing school for practice as a nurse.

22 Louise L. Hay, 1996, Heal Your Body: the Mental Causes for Physical Illness and the Metaphysical Way to Overcome Them, Carlsbad, CA: Hay House

23 "A Quote by Heraclitus," Goodreads. Goodreads,
Accessed October 1, 2019, https://www.goodreads.com/
quotes/336994-the-only-thing-that-is-constant-is-change--

24 Author's Note: Adrenal fatigue is a functional term and not recognized as a
medical diagnosis and has no ICD classification/fee code. Because the adrenal
glands do not actually stop functioning, this is looked at medically as more
of a dysfunctional state called HPA-D (hypothalamus-pituitary-adrenal axis
dysfunction) of which the symptoms are treated with drugs to elevate mood,
cause sleep, or stimulate attention. None of these address the cause which
is more difficult to identify and treat. That requires self care, sleep hygiene,
diet modifications, lifestyle changes, herbal supplements, detoxification, and
supplementation with micro-nutrient replacement of building blocks for
neurotransmitters, hormones and cellular energy.

25 T. H. Holmes, and R. H. Rahe, N.D., "The Social Readjustment Rating Scale,"
Garfield Library, University of Pennsylvania, Accessed May 5, 2019. http://www.
garfield.library.upenn.edu/classics1982/A1982PJ13900001.pdf
Originally published in The Week's Citation Classic 11:213-12, 1967,
Department of Psychiatry, University of Washington School of Medicine.

26 Scott Jeffery, "Understanding Your Level of Consciousness: How to
Raise It." *The Healers Journal*, www.thehealersjournal.com/2013/07/26/
hawkins-scale-consciousness-how-to-raise-your-number/

27 Catharine Paddock, PhD, 2012, "Smiling Reduces Stress And Helps The Heart."
Medical News Today, MediLexicon International, August 1, 2012, https://www.
medicalnewstoday.com/articles/248433.php

28 Han Selye, 1946, "The General Adaptation Syndrome and the Diseases
of Adaptation," JACI Online, The Journal of Allergy and Clinical
Immunology, Accessed May 11, 2018, https://www.jacionline.org/
article/0021-8707(46)90148-7/fulltext

29 Ott, Martin, et al. Mitochondria, Oxidative Stress and Cell Death. Apoptosis
(2007) 12:913–922, 9 Feb. 2007, link.springer.com/content/pdf/10.1007/
s10495-007-0756-2.pdf, DOI 10.1007/s10495-007-0756-2

30 Author comment: This table is intended to facilitate general understanding of
information and is presented as a suggested comparison, for illustration purposes
in the context of this book only. No medical, psychological, legal or other claims
intended.

31 "Depletions to Renewal Grid." *Building Personal Resilience: HeartMath Skills for
Personal Effectiveness*, Institute of HeartMath, 2014, pp. 8–10

32 Alyssa W. Goldman, Yvonne Burmeister, Konstantin Cesnulevicius, Martha
Herbert, Mary Kane, David Lescheid, Timothy McCaffrey, et al, 2015,
"Bioregulatory Systems Medicine: an Innovative Approach to Integrating the
Science of Molecular Networks, Inflammation, and Systems Biology with the
Patient's Autoregulatory Capacity?" Frontiers in Physiology, Frontiers Media S.A.
August 19, 2015, https://www.ncbi.nlm.nih.gov/pmc/articles/PMC4541032/

33 Smit, Alta, Arturo O'Byrne, Bruno Van Brandt, Ivo Bianchi, and Klaus
Kuestermann. 2010. "Disease Development." Alternative & Complementary
Therapies 16 (3). https://www.hoffmancentre.com/wp-content/uploads/pdfs/ama/
Disease_Development.pdf

34 Homotoxicology Disease Evolution Table, BioPathica Limited, 28 May 2018,
www.biopathica.co.uk/6%20Phases%20Of%20Disease.htm

"Homotoxicology" being the study of the impact of toxins on humans; and the DET an instrument allowing for the evaluation of disease progression.

35 Naviaux, Robert K. "Metabolic Features of the Cell Danger Response." Elsevier, 24 Aug. 2013, www.elsevier.com/ locate/mito, by Elsevier B.V. and Mitochondria Research Society

36 Daniel Goleman, Emotional Intelligence, New York: Bantam Books, 2006

37 Herbert Benson and Miriam Z. Klipper, 2000, The Relaxation Response, New York: Harper

38 "About." Candace Pert, PhD, Candace Pert, PhD , candacepert.com/, Accessed October 12, 2018

Endnotes - Chapter 5

1 Cody Delistraty, 2019, "The Intelligence of Plants." *The Paris Review*, September 30, 2019, https://www.theparisreview.org/blog/2019/09/26/ the-intelligence-of-plants/?utm_source=pocket-newtab

2 Mudra V. Bhatt, Aditi Khandelwal, and Susan A. Dudley, 2010, "Kin Recognition, Not Competitive Interactions, Predicts Root Allocation in Young Cakile Edentula Seedling Pairs," *New Phytologist Trust*, John Wiley & Sons, Ltd (10.1111), November 30, 2010 https://nph.onlinelibrary.wiley.com/ doi/10.1111/j.1469-8137.2010.03548.x

3 Han Selye, 1946, "The General Adaptation Syndrome and the Diseases of Adaptation," JACI Online, The Journal of Allergy and Clinical Immunology, Accessed May 11, 2018, https://www.jacionline.org/ article/0021-8707(46)90148-7/fulltext

4 Kendra Cherry, 2019, "Why Optimal Arousal Levels Lead to Better Athletic Performance," Verywell Mind, June 15, 2019, https://www.verywellmind.com/ what-is-the-yerkes-dodson-law-2796027

5 Amy Arnsten, F T, 2009, "Stress Signalling Pathways That Impair Prefrontal Cortex Structure and Function," Nature Reviews, Neuroscience, U.S. National Library of Medicine, June 2009, https://www.ncbi.nlm.nih.gov/pmc/articles/ PMC2907136/, https://dx.doi.org/10.1038/nrn2648

6 "Thomas Jefferson Quotes." n.d. BrainyQuote. Xplore. Accessed December 13, 2019. https://www.brainyquote.com/quotes/thomas_jefferson_132201

7 "Joyce Carol Oates Teaches the Art of the Short Story," n.d., MasterClass Advertisement, MasterClass, Accessed December 3, 2019, https://www. masterclass.com/classes/joyce-carol-oates-teaches-the-art-of-the-short-story

8 Brenner, MD FAPA, Grant Hilary. 2018. "Your Brain on Creativity." Psychology Today. Sussex Publishers. February 22, 2018. https://www.psychologytoday.com/ us/blog/experimentations/201802/your-brain-creativity

9 Beaty RE, Kenett YN, Christensen AP, Rosenberg MD, Benedek M, Chen Q, Fink A, Qiu J, Kwapil TR, Kane MJ & Silva PJ. "Robust prediction of individual creative ability from brain functional connectivity." PNAS 2018 January, 115 (5) 1087-1092. https://doi.org/10.1073/pnas.1713532115

10 Reporter, 2015,"The True Story behind 'The Cranky Old Man' Internet Poem That Has Become World Famous," Sunday Post, December 7, 2015,

https://www.sundaypost.com/news/uk-news/the-true-story-behind-the-cranky-old-man-internet-poem-that-has-become-world-famous/
Author's note: This poem has sometimes been published as "Look Closer," "Look Closer Nurse," "Kate," "Open Your Eyes," "A Crabbit Old Woman," or "What Do You See?" I found that its history and poet author can be confused with "The Cranky Old Man." Also there appear to be several versions. This is the version that I have and I include it here because it is the one that inspired me. However, it is attributed to Anonymous and is a little longer than the version from The Sunday Post from the United Kingdom.

11 Tvaraj, 2013, "David L. Griffith," Impressions, August 27, 2013, https://tvaraj. com/tag/david-l-griffith/
Contains information reproduced from a letter from the son of Phyllis McCormick claiming her to be the original author who submitted the poem anonymously to a the magazine for Sunnyside Hospital. In Scottish, Crabbit means "bad-tempered" or "grumpy".

12 Girija Kaimal, Kendra Ray and Juan Muniz, 2016, "Reduction of Cortisol Levels and Participants' Responses Following Art Making," Art Therapy, 33:2, 74-80, DOI: 10.1080/07421656.2016.1166832, https://www.tandfonline.com/doi/full/10.1080/07421656.2016.1166832

13 Teresa M. Amabile and Steven J. Kramer, "Time Pressure and Creativity." *The Progress Principle*, Harvard Business Press, 2011, pp. 106–108.

14 "Flow (Psychology)." *Wikipedia*, Wikimedia Foundation, 13 Dec. 2018, en.wikipedia.org/wiki/Flow (psychology).

15 "Paradigm - Dictionary Definition." Vocabulary.com, Accessed October 26, 2019, https://www.vocabulary.com/dictionary/paradigm

16 Strate, Cody. 2018. "How Does Patient Satisfaction Impact Reimbursement?" How Does Patient Satisfaction Impact Reimbursement? March 20, 2018. https://www.accessefm.com/blog/how-does-patient-satisfaction-impact-reimbursement

17 Mark J. Perry, 2017, "Health Care Is a Commodity, Not a Right – and Markets, Not Government Are the Solution in Medical Care." AEI. January 13, 2017, https://www.aei.org/carpe-diem/health-care-is-a-commodity-not-a-right-and-markets-not-government-are-the-solution-in-medical-care/

18 Saad, Lydia. "U.S. Ethics Ratings Rise for Medical Workers and Teachers." Gallup. com, Gallup, 23 Mar. 2021, news.gallup.com/poll/328136/ethics-ratings-rise-medical-workers-teachers.aspx

19 Riane Eisler and Lucy Garrick. "Leading the Shift from a Dominator to a Partnership Culture." *The Systems Thinker*, 6 Feb. 2018, thesystemsthinker.com/leading-the-shift-from-a-dominator-to-a-partnership-culture/

20 Serusha Govender, "Nocebo Effect: How Negative Thinking Affects Your Health," WebMD, WebMD, Accessed June 13, 2019, https://www.webmd.com/balance/features/is-the-nocebo-effect-hurting-your-health#1
"...a sort of negative placebo effect called the nocebo effect. It's what happens when you're given a sugar pill, are told it's a drug that has terrible side effects, then start to exhibit those symptoms... Just knowing the risks could negatively impact your recovery... all because of the power of suggestion... The Verdict: If you believe a treatment won't help you, it probably won't -- and vice versa."

21 Sheldon Cohen, "The Perceived Stres Scale," NH Department of Administrative Services, das.nh.gov/wellness/docs/percieved%20stress%20scale.pdf

22 Watanabe, Jonathan H., Terry McInnis, and Jan D. Hirsch. 2018. "Cost of

Prescription Drug–Related Morbidity and Mortality - Jonathan H. Watanabe, Terry McInnis, Jan D. Hirsch, 2018." SAGE Journals. September 2018. https://journals.sagepub.com/doi/abs/10.1177/1060028018765159

23   "Niels Bohr Quotes," n.d. BrainyQuote, Xplore, Accessed May 19, 2019, https://www.brainyquote.com/quotes/niels_bohr_164546

24   Quora. 2017. "What Is A Quantum Field, And How Does It Interact With Matter?" Forbes. Forbes Magazine. December 20, 2017. https://www.forbes.com/sites/quora/2017/12/20/what-is-a-quantum-field-and-how-does-it-interact-with-matter/#3ca409f828c4

25   Ajeshkumar Kumar, 2015, "NURSING THEORY Martha Rogers - The Science of Unitary Human Beings," LinkedIn SlideShare, MM College of Nursing, MM University Mullana, Ambala, Haryana, India, April 20, 2015, https://www.slideshare.net/ajeshktk/subh-martha

26   Ross, Christina L. 2019. "Energy Medicine: Current Status and Future Perspectives." Global Advances in Health and Medicine. SAGE Publications. February 27, 2019. https://www.ncbi.nlm.nih.gov/pmc/articles/PMC6396053/

27   ibid

28   Goodson, Scott. 2014. "Warren Berger Tells How to Ask a 'Beautiful Question'." The Daily Beast. The Daily Beast Company. March 8, 2014. https://www.thedailybeast.com/warren-berger-tells-how-to-ask-a-beautiful-question

29   "Shunryu Suzuki Quotes (Author of Zen Mind, Beginner's Mind)," n.d. Goodreads.com, Goodreads, Accessed November 23, 2019, https://www.goodreads.com/work/quotes/231282-zen-mind-beginner-s-mind

Endnotes - Chapter 6

1   Rollin McCraty, PhD, "The Energetic Heart: Biolectromagnetic Interactions Within and Between People." Research Gate, July 2003, Accessed December 18, 2018, https://www.researchgate.net/publication/274451622_The_Energetic_Heart_Biolectromagnetic_Interactions_Within_and_Between_People, 1.

2   ibid

3   Rollin McCraty, PhD, "Heart-brain Communication," Science of Heart: Exploring the Role of the Heart in Human Performance, 3. Vol. 2. Boulder Creek, CA: HearthMath Institute, 2015

4   "Bioelectronic Medicine – Speaking the Body's Electrical Language," Pharmaceutical Technology, September 18, 2013, Accessed November 20, 2018, https://www.pharmaceutical-technology.com/features/feature-bioelectronic-medicine-body-electrical-language-gsk/

5   Michael Behar, "Can the Nervous System Be Hacked?" The New York Times, The New York Times, 23 May 2014, www.nytimes.com/2014/05/25/magazine/can-the-nervous-system-be-hacked.html

6   "Meditation: In Depth," *National Center for Complementary and Integrative Health*, January 02, 2019, Accessed June 16, 2019, https://nccih.nih.gov/health/meditation/overview.htm

7   Richard J. Davidson, Jon Kabat-Zinn, Jessica Schumacher, Melissa Rosenkranz, Daniel Muller, Saki F. Santorelli, Ferris Urbanowski, Anne Harrington, Katherine Bonus, and John F. Sheridan. "Alterations in Brain and Immune Function

Produced by Mindfulness Meditation," *Psychosomatic Medicine,* 2003, Accessed June 16, 2019, https://www.ncbi.nlm.nih.gov/pubmed/12883106

8   "9 Fascinating Facts About the Vagus Nerve." Mental Floss, Mental Floss, 13 Nov. 2018, mentalfloss.com/article/65710/9-nervy-facts-about-vagus-nerve . New research has revealed that it may also be the missing link to treating chronic inflammation, and the beginning of an exciting new field of treatment for serious, incurable diseases.

9   Gidron, Yori, Reginald Deschepper, Marijke De Couck, Julian F Thayer, and Brigitte Velkeniers. 2018. "The Vagus Nerve Can Predict and Possibly Modulate Non-Communicable Chronic Diseases: Introducing a Neuroimmunological Paradigm to Public Health." Journal of Clinical Medicine. MDPI. October 19, 2018. https://www.ncbi.nlm.nih.gov/pmc/articles/PMC6210465/ , doi: 10.3390/jcm7100371.

10   Howland, Robert H. 2014. "Vagus Nerve Stimulation." Current Behavioral Neuroscience Reports. U.S. National Library of Medicine. June 2014. https://www.ncbi.nlm.nih.gov/pmc/articles/PMC4017164/, doi: 10.1007/s40473-014-0010-5.

11   Marijke De Couck, Ralf Caers, David Spiegel, and Yori Gidron, "The Role of the Vagus Nerve in Cancer Prognosis: A Systematic and a Comprehensive Review." *Journal of Oncology,* July 02, 2018, Accessed July 14, 2018, https://www.ncbi.nlm.nih.gov/pmc/articles/PMC6051067/

12   "Infinity Symbol," n.d., Infinity Symbol (blog), Accessed July 27, 2019, https://www.infinitysymbol.net/
     The infinity symbol (∞) looks like a horizontal version of number 8. As a line that never ends, it represents the concept of eternity, endless, unlimited and everlasting. It was first used by Wallis in the mid 1650's in the context of mathematics, but has also found usefulness in physics and metaphysics.

13   McCraty, Rollin, Mike Atkinson, and Raymond Trevor Bradley. 2004. "Electrophysiological Evidence of Intuition: Part 1. The Surprising Role of the Heart," Journal of Alternative and Complementary Medicine (New York, N.Y.). U.S. National Library of Medicine. February 2004. https://www.ncbi.nlm.nih.gov/pubmed/15025887

14   McCraty, Rollin, Mike Atkinson, and Raymond Trevor Bradley. 2004. "Electrophysiological Evidence of Intuition: Part 2. A System-Wide Process?" Journal of Alternative and Complementary Medicine (New York, N.Y.). U.S. National Library of Medicine. April 2004. https://www.ncbi.nlm.nih.gov/pubmed/15165413

Endnotes - Chapter 7

1   Steve Tobak, "The Value of Stick-with-It-Ness." CBS News, CBS Interactive, 7 July 2009, www.cbsnews.com/news/the-value-of-stick-with-it-ness/
     Author Comment: One of two similar phrases found on an internet search for the phrase used in this book: "Stick-to-it-ness" used by my Mom that guided me to develop courage and stamina to see things through. Steve Tobak says, "As I define it, Stick-with-It-Ness, means perseverance in the face of extraordinary competition, determination against long odds, optimism when everyone else has thrown in the towel, and standing up after being knocked down again and again."

2   "Stick-to-Itiveness," *Merriam-Webster*, Merriam Webster www.merriam-webster.com/dictionary/stick-to-itiveness "Stick-to-itiveness" is tenacity. First known use

was in 1859. Author comment: This is one of two similar phrases found on an internet search for the phrase used in this book, "Stick-to-it-ness" used by my Mom that guided me to develop courage and stamina to see things through.

3   Toby Keith, As Good As I Once Was, Toby Keith, Recorded 2004, James Stroud; Toby Keith, CD. Written by Toby Keith and Scotty Emerick, Label- DreamWorks Nashville, Album -Honkytonk University album

4   "A Quote by Frank Zappa," n.d., Goodreads, Goodreads, Accessed January 19, 2020, https://www.goodreads.com/ quotes/33052-a-mind-is-like-a-parachute-it-doesn-t-work-if

5   Irving Berlin, "Irving Berlin Quotes," BrainyQuote, Xplore, www.brainyquote. com/quotes/irving_berlin_116687

6   Brian Tracy, 2018, "The Power of Your Subconscious Mind," Brian Tracy's Self Improvement & Professional Development Blog, Brian Tracy International Publisher Logo, December 12, 2018, https://www.briantracy.com/blog/ personal-success/understanding-your-subconscious-mind/

7   "Insanity Is Doing the Same Thing Over and Over Again and Expecting Different Results," Quote Investigator, Quoteinvestigator.com/2017/03/23/same/ Source unknown though often attributed to Einstein.

8   "The Science of HeartMath," 2019, HeartMath, June 13, 2019, https://www. heartmath.com/science/

9   Arlin Cuncic, 2019, "How to Prevent and Cope From an Amygdala Hijack," Verywell Mind, Verywell Mind, August 18, 2019, https://www.verywellmind. com/what-happens-during-an-amygdala-hijack-4165944

10   Depak Chopra, "Seven Myths of Meditation." DeepakChopra.com, Accessed June 19, 2019. https://www.deepakchopra.com/blog/article/4275

11   Buczynski, Dr. Ruth, and Bruce Lipton. The National Institute for the Clinical Application of Behavioral Medicine, www.nicabm.com "How Epigenetics Can Change Your View of the Mind and the Spirit." The National Institute for the Clinical Application of Behavioral Medicine. Transcribed Teleseminar Interview. Accessed May 05,2019. www.itineriscoaching.com/wp-content/uploads/2011/03/ Epigenetics-Bruce-Lipton.pdf

12   Harvard Health Publishing. "The Power of the Placebo Effect." Harvard Health . Harvard Health Publishing (Harvard Medical School), May 2017. https://www. health.harvard.edu/mental-health/the-power-of-the-placebo-effect

13   Fabrizio Benedetti, Claudia Arduino, Sara Costa, Sergio Vighetti, Luisella Tarenzi, Innocenzo Rainero, and Giovanni Asteggiano, "Loss of Expectation-related Mechanisms in Alzheimer's Disease Makes Analgesic Therapies Less Effective," Pain, March 2006, Accessed November 03, 2018, https://www.ncbi.nlm.nih.gov/ pubmed/16473462/

14   Damien G. Finniss, Ted J Kaptchuk, Franklin Miller, and Fabrizio Benedetti, 2010, "Biological, Clinical, and Ethical Advances of Placebo Effects," The Lancet 375 (9715): 686–95, https://doi.org/10.1016/s0140-6736(09)61706-2

15   Lissa Rankin, MD, "Is There Scientific Proof We Can Heal Ourselves?" 2012, TEDxAmericanRiviera, August 15, 2012, https://tedxamericanriviera.com/ lissa-rankin-md-is-there-scientific-proof-we-can-heal-ourselves/

16   Lipton, Bruce, PhD and Ruth Buczynski, PhD "How Eigentics Can Change Your View of the Mind and the Spirit." Teleseminar. Featuring Dr. Bruce Lipton.

The complete transcript of a teleseminar featuring Dr. Bruce Lipton, and conducted by Dr Ruth Buczynski of NICABM, Accessed June 19, 2019 https://www.slideshare.net/liberleon/bruce-lipton-epigenetics, 10.

17   Xue Zheng, Ryan Fehr, Kenneth Tai, Jayanth Narayanan, Michele J. Gelfand, (2014), "The Unburdening Effects of Forgiveness: Effects on Slant Perception and Jumping Height," *Social Psychological and Personality Science*, 6. 431-438, https://journals.sagepub.com/doi/10.1177/1948550614564222

18   "A Quote by Thomas A. Edison," Goodreads, Goodreads, www.goodreads.com/quotes/13639-the-doctor-of-the-future-will-give-no-medication-but

Endnotes - Chapter 8

1   Holden, Robert. "Shift Happens!: Powerful Ways to Transform Your Life." Hay House, 2010.

2   Tania Luna and Jordan Cohen, 2018, "To Get People to Change, Make Change Easy," Harvard Business Review, May 14, 2018, https://hbr.org/2017/12/to-get-people-to-change-make-change-easy

3   Holden, Robert. "Shift Happens!: Powerful Ways to Transform Your Life." Hay House, 2010.

4   *A Course in Miracles*, (Glen Elen, CA: Foundation for Inner Peace, 1985). Text 10:573.
    Text is of three books that is a sections in the combined book, Chapter 10 in that book/section and page 573.

5   Dan Millman, *Way of the Peaceful Warrior*, (H.J. Kramer, 2006)
    Authors' note: I was unable to locate the publisher for the 1980 version that I had and regretfully no longer own. This is the revised edition.

6   Leon F. Seltzer, 2016. "You Only Get More of What You Resist-Why?" Psychology Today, Sussex Publishers, June 15, 2016, https://www.psychologytoday.com/us/blog/evolution-the-self/201606/you-only-get-more-what-you-resist-why

7   "Elisabeth Kubler-Ross Quotes," n.d., BrainyQuote, Xplore, Accessed May 23, 2018, https://www.brainyquote.com/quotes/elisabeth_kublerross_119810

Endnotes - Chapter 9

1   Steve Jobs, "Steve Jobs Quotes," BrainyQuote, Accessed November 26, 2018, https://www.brainyquote.com/quotes/steve_jobs_416875

2   Author note: To thrive means to flourish or grow vigorously which cannot happen when the survival mechanisms of fight or flight are activated. I use the word thrival, which may differ from others' usage, to refer to an attainable to which we can aspire state beyond mere survival. This is in contrast to the survival mechanisms and skills like inflammation, fight or flight, bobbing for air while treading water or living paycheck-to-paycheck, which are energy depleting and unsustainable. Thrival skills help attain and maintain abundant energy, joy, health and vibrancy which include expressing virtues of serenity, courage, presence, creativity and flow.

3   Steven P. Hams, 2000, "A Gut Feeling? Intuition and Critical Care Nursing," Intensive & Critical Care Nursing, U.S. National Library of Medicine, October 2000, https://www.ncbi.nlm.nih.gov/pubmed/11000605

4   Deborah Binder, "Counting Thoughts, Part I," Exploring the Problem Space, Exploring the Problem Space, January 1, 2017, https://www.exploringtheproblemspace.com/new-blog/2017/1/1/counting-thoughts-part-i

5   Stephanie Liou, "Meditation and HD," HOPES Huntington's Disease Information, July 27, 2016, https://hopes.stanford.edu/meditation-and-hd/

6   Edwards, Lin. 2010. "Study Suggests Reliance on GPS May Reduce Hippocampus Function as We Age." Medical Xpress - Medical Research Advances and Health News. Medical Xpress. November 18, 2010. https://medicalxpress.com/news/2010-11-reliance-gps-hippocampus-function-age.html

7   Harvard Health Publishing. 2018. "Takotsubo Cardiomyopathy (Broken-Heart Syndrome)." Harvard Health. April 2, 2018. https://www.health.harvard.edu/heart-health/takotsubo-cardiomyopathy-broken-heart-syndrome

8   Author note: Hospitals and facilities have code names for incidents that may occur. "Code blue" is commonly used for a life threatening medical situation, usually involving the impairment or cessation of someone's breathing or heart beat. Traditionally it was the most emergent situation and became known as "a code" for short. The "code team" is usually a team of staff members who respond to the code call, arriving with medications, equipment and expertise.

9   Merriam-Webster. Merriam-Webster. Accessed February 4, 2020. https://www.merriam-webster.com/dictionary/stat [As used in medicine] Without delay; immediately [often emergent]

10   Author note: "Crash" is a term used by nurses and medical staff that refers to the condition of a patient declining rapidly and precipitously.

Endnotes - Chapter 10

1   Kabat-Zinn, Jon. 2013. Full Catastrophe Living, Revised Edition: How to Cope with Stress, Pain and Illness Using Mindfulness Meditation. United Kingdom: Piatkus, p 99

2   The Virtues Project was founded in Canada in 1991 by Linda Kavelin-Popov, Dr. Dan Popov and John Kavelin. It's a global grassroots initiative to inspire the practice of virtues in everyday life. It was honored by the United Nations during the International Year of the Family as a "model global program for families of all cultures". https://virtuesproject.com/

3   "Zen & the Japanese Arts." n.d. Zen and Japanese Arts | Zen Buddhism. Accessed October 29, 2019. https://www.zenlightenment.net/arts/zen-and-arts.html

4   Ibid

5   Chevalier, Sinatra, Stephen T., Oschman, James L., Sokal, Karol, Sokal, and Pawel, 2012, "Earthing: Health Implications of Reconnecting the Human Body to the Earth's Surface Electrons," Journal of Environmental and Public Health, Hindawi, January 12, 2012, https://www.hindawi.com/journals/jeph/2012/291541/

6   For Love of the Game, Directed by Sam Raimi, Performed by Kevin Costner, United States: Universal Pictures, 1999, Film, https://www.imdb.com/title/

tt0126916/characters/nm0000126
Kevin Costner's character, Billy Chapel's trick for concentration: Clear the
mechanism. https://www.youtube.com/watch?v=aXrpmN6hHqc

7   "Well (n.)." n.d. Index. Accessed April 8, 2019. https://www.etymonline.com/
     word/well#etymonline_v_7908
     Comment: Century Dictionary

Endnotes - Chapter 11

1   "Well: Search Online Etymology Dictionary." n.d. Index. Accessed April 8, 2019.
     https://www.etymonline.com/search?q=well
     Comment: Gothic adv. "to wish, will;" Old English v. "to spring, rise, gush;" Old
     English n. "spring of water, fountain," "source"

2   "Well (Adv.)." n.d. Index. Accessed April 8, 2019. https://www.etymonline.com/
     word/well#etymonline_v_7908
     Comment: Old English v. "to wish, desire;" Germanic v. "to wish, will;" Sanskrit
     vrnoti v. "chooses;" "according to one's wish;" wela "well-being, riches;" Old
     English, "The implication of intention or volition distinguishes it from shall,
     which expresses or implies obligation or necessity."

3   Dossey, Larry. 2006. The Extraordinary Healing Power of Ordinary Things:
     Fourteen Natural Steps to Health and Happiness. New York: Harmony Books.

4   "A Quote by Miguel Ruiz." n.d. Goodreads. Goodreads.
     Accessed December 4, 2019. https://www.goodreads.com/
     quotes/71463-1-be-impeccable-with-your-word-speak-with-integrity-say

5   "Law of Attraction (New Thought)," Wikipedia, Accessed June 29, 2019. https://
     en.wikipedia.org/wiki/Law_of_attraction_(New_Thought).
     In this philosophy, the belief is that positive or negative thoughts respectively
     bring positive or negative experiences into a person's life. It is based on the idea
     that people and their thoughts are vibratory in nature and made from pure energy,
     and that through the process of resonance, like energy attracting like energy, a
     person can improve their own health, wealth, and personal relationships.

6   "You Can't Afford the Luxury of a Negative Thought" by Peter McWilliams
     - Paperback: HarperCollins. 2001. HarperCollins UK. HarperCollins
     Publishers. April 2, 2001. https://www.harpercollins.co.uk/9780007107568/
     you-cant-afford-the-luxury-of-a-negative-thought/

7   aad, Lydia. "U.S. Ethics Ratings Rise for Medical Workers and Teachers." Gallup.
     com, Gallup, 23 Mar. 2021, news.gallup.com/poll/328136/ethics-ratings-rise-
     medical-workers-teachers.aspx

8   Committee on the RWJF Initiative on the Future of Nursing, "The Future of
     Nursing: Leading Change, Advancing Health" - NACNS, Accessed May 6, 2018,
     http://www.nacns.org/wp-content/uploads/2016/11/5-IOM-Report.pdf

9   Tony Fahkry, "Why The Purpose For Your Life Is To Experience
     The Fullness Of Who You Really Are." Tony Fahkry (blog), January
     29, 2019, Accessed January 30, 2019, http://www.tonyfahkry.com/
     why-the-purpose-for-your-life-is-to-experience-the-fullness-of-who-you-really-are/

10   "A Quote by National Library Week." Goodreads, Goodreads, www.goodreads.
     com/quotes/576292-the-more-you-read-the-more-you-know-the-more

Endnotes - Chapter 12

1   Rick Hanson, 2014, Hardwiring Happiness: the Practical Science of Reshaping Your Brain and Your Life, London: Rider Books

2   David B. Yaden, Jonathan Iwry, Johannes C. Eiechstaedt, George E. Vaillant, Kelley J. Slack, Yukun Zhao, and Andrew B. Newberg, 2016, "The Overview Effect: Awe and Self-Transcendent Experience in Space Flight." AndrewNewberg. com, American Psychoiogical Association. 2016. http://www.andrewnewberg. com/s/the-overview-effect.pdf, http://dx.doi.org/10.1037/cns0000086

3   "Awe," Dictionary.com, Dictionary.com, Accessed October 24, 2019, https://www. dictionary.com/browse/awe
    Awe is an overwhelming feeling of reverence, admiration, fear, etc., produced by that which is grand, sublime, extremely powerful, or the like.

4   "Transcendent," Dictionary.com, Dictionary.com, Accessed October 24, 2019, https://www.dictionary.com/browse/transcendent
    The quality or state of going beyond ordinary limits; surpassing; exceeding.

5   Andrew B. Newberg and Mark Robert Waldman, 2016, "How Enlightenment Changes Your Brain: The New Science of Transformation," Avery.

6   Alex Korb,PhD, 2011, "Boosting Your Serotonin Activity," Psychology Today, Sussex Publishers, November 17, 2011, https://www.psychologytoday.com/us/ blog/prefrontal-nudity/201111/boosting-your-serotonin-activity

7   Tiffany Field, Maria Hernandez-Reif, Miguel Diego, Saul Schanberg, and Cynthia Kuhn, 2005,"Cortisol Decreases and Serotonin and Dopamine Increase Following Massage Therapy," The International Journal of Neuroscience, U.S. National Library of Medicine, October 2005, https://www.ncbi.nlm.nih.gov/ pubmed/16162447

8   Saad, Lydia. "U.S. Ethics Ratings Rise for Medical Workers and Teachers." Gallup. com, Gallup, 23 Mar. 2021, news.gallup.com/poll/328136/ethics-ratings-rise-medical-workers-teachers.aspx

9   Zane, J. Peder. 2012. "Imaginary Prizes Take Aim at Real Problems." The New York Times. The New York Times. November 9, 2012

10 Ibid

11 Warren Berger Author. n.d. "Why Should You Care About Questioning? - A More Beautiful Question by Warren Berger." A More Beautiful Question by Warren Berger. Accessed November 8, 2019. https://amorebeautifulquestion.com/ why-should-you-care/

12 Michelle Griffin, and Ardeshir Bayat. "Electrical Stimulation in Bone Healing: Critical Analysis by Evaluating Levels of Evidence." Pub Med, U.S. National Library of Medicine, pubmed.ncbi.nlm.nih.gov/21847434/.Eplasty. 2011;11:e34. Epub 2011 Jul 26. PMID: 21847434; PMCID: PMC3145421

13 Ott, Martin, et al. Mitochondria, Oxidative Stress and Cell Death. Apoptosis (2007) 12:913–922, 9 Feb. 2007, link.springer.com/content/pdf/10.1007/s10495-007-0756-2.pdf
    DOI 10.1007/s10495-007-0756-2

14 Lynne McTaggert, 2002, "The Field" (ebook), Accessed September 8, 2019, https://universeisathought.files.wordpress.com/2014/11/the-field.pdf, Harper Collins, New York, Prologue, VIII: Human beings and all living things are a coalescence of energy in a field of energy connected to every other thing in the

world. This pulsating energy field is the central engine of our being and our consciousness, …There is no 'me' and 'not-me' duality to our bodies in relation to the uni-verse, but one underlying energy field. This field is responsible for our mind's highest functions, the information source guiding the growth of our bodies. It is our brain, our heart, our memory – indeed, a blueprint of the world for all time. The field is the force, rather than germs or genes,

15 Morgan, Jacob. 2017. "A Simple Explanation Of 'The Internet Of Things'." Forbes. Forbes Magazine. April 20, 2017. https://www.forbes.com/sites/jacobmorgan/2014/05/13/ simple-explanation-internet-things-that-anyone-can-understand/#327a86c91d09

16 "Emanation," Emanation Definition - Google Search, Accessed September 9, 2019, https://bit.ly/2lFWAal noun: 1. an abstract but perceptible thing that issues or originates from a source. 2. the action or process of issuing from a source.

17 JohnMark Taylor. "Mirror Neurons After a Quarter Century: New Light, New Cracks." Science in the News, 15 Aug. 2016, sitn.hms.harvard.edu/flash/2016/ mirror-neurons-quarter-century-new-light-new-cracks/

Original discovery research, Understanding motor events: A neurophysiological study published February 1992 in Experimental Brain Research 91(1):176-80 DOI:10.1007/BF00230027

18 Nadeau, Robert, and Minas C. Kafatos. "The Non-Local Universe: the New Physics and Matters of the Mind". Oxford University Press, 2001, p 97

19 M. Capek, "The Philosophical Impact of Contemporary Physics", Princeton, NJ, D. Van Nostrand, 1961): 319, as quoted by Tom McFarland, 2015, Quora (blog), https://www.quora.com/ Where-did-Einstein-write-that-the-field-is-the-only-reality

20 Kelly, Megan. "How Prayer Changes the Brain and Body Prayer Changes the Brain." Renewing All Things, 8 Feb. 2018, renewingallthings.com/ spiritual-health/how-prayer-changes-the-brain-and-body/

21 "GCI." HeartMath Institute, www.heartmath.org/gci/ The GCI seeks to help activate the heart of humanity and promote peace, harmony and a shift in global consciousness.

22 Gregg Braden, "World's magnetic field changed immediately after 9/11," published on Apr 27, 2015, YouTube, https://youtu.be/70Wi4YIkpmk, 2:17 – 2:42

23 Hawkins, David R., M. D., Ph D., Power vs. Force: the Hidden Determinants of Human Behavior: Author's Official Authoritative Edition. Hay House Inc, 2014.

24 "Power of 10," 2019, Wikipedia, Wikimedia Foundation, September 26, 2019, https://en.wikipedia.org/wiki/Power_of_10

25 Hawkins, David R., M. D., Ph D., "Power vs. Force: the Hidden Determinants of Human Behavior: Author's Official Authoritative Edition". Hay House Inc, 2014.

Endnotes - Chapter 13

1 Hendricks, Scotty. 2019. "Is Your Negativity Getting in the Way of Your Creativity?" Big Think. Big Think. January 30, 2019. https://bigthink.com/ good-news-you-can-overcome-negativity-bias

2 Peter McWilliams, You Can't Afford the Luxury of a Negative Thought (The

Life 101 Series) 1985, Luxury Quotes, Accessed September 27, 2019, http://
petermcwilliams.org/page198.html

3   A Course in Miracles. 1992. Glen Elen, CA: Foundation for Inner Peace.
Lesson 34: https://acim.org/workbook/lesson-34/

4   Fawcett, Jacqueline. " ROGERS' SCIENCE OF UNITARY HUMAN BEINGS:
AN OVERVIEW." SOCIETYOFROGERIANSCHOLARS.ORG, www.
societyofrogerianscholars.org/about.html
Synoptic overview of Martha E. Rogers' conceptual system, the Science of Unitary
Human Beings, including the definition: Integrality is defined as the "continuous
mutual human [energy] field and environmental [energy] field process (Rogers,
1990, p. 8) that characterizes the nature of the integral and indivisible relationship
between the human and environmental energy fields."

Endnotes - Chapter 14

1   Toney-Butler, Tammy J. 2019. "Nursing Process." StatPearls [Internet]. U.S.
National Library of Medicine. July 30, 2019. https://www.ncbi.nlm.nih.gov/
books/NBK499937/

2   Rubinstein, J. S., Meyer, D. E. & Evans, J. E. (2001). "Executive Control of
Cognitive Processes in Task Switching." Journal of Experimental Psychology:
Human Perception and Performance, 27, 763-797

3   "Multitasking: Switching Costs - Subtle 'Switching' Costs Cut Efficiency, Raise
Risk." American Psychological Association, American Psychological Association,
20 Mar. 2006, www.apa.org/research/action/multitask

4   Mariotti, Agnese. "The Effects of Chronic Stress on Health: New Insights into
the Molecular Mechanisms of Brain-Body Communication." Future Science
OA, Future Science Ltd, 1 Nov. 2015, www.ncbi.nlm.nih.gov/pmc/articles/
PMC5137920/

5   "The Ed Sullivan Show," The Plate Spinner - Erich Brenn, Co-created and
produced by Mario Lewis, season 21, episode 18, Columbia Broadcasting System
(CBS) -TV Studio 50, 16 Feb. 1969,
View video online: https://www.youtube.com/watch?v=Zhoos1oY404 Other
citation information sources: https://www.metacritic.com/tv/the-ed-sullivan-
show/season-21/episode-18-february-16-1969-blood-sweat-tears-caterina-valente-
arthur-godfrey and https://en.wikipedia.org/wiki/The_Ed_Sullivan_Show

6   Marcel Schwantes, 2018, "Warren Buffett Says This 1 Simple Habit Separates
Successful People From Everyone Else," Inc.com, Inc. January 18, 2018, https://
www.inc.com/marcel-schwantes/warren-buffett-says-this-is-1-simple-habit-that-
separates-successful-people-from-everyone-else

Endnotes - Chapter 15

1   Garson, n.d. "Whether You Believe You Can Do a Thing or Not, You Are
Right," Quote Investigator, Accessed June 11, 2018, https://quoteinvestigator.
com/2015/02/03/you-can/

2   Star Wars Episode V: The Empire Strikes Back. Directed by Irvin Kershner. Story
by Lucas Geroge. Screenplay by Lawrence Kasdan. Performed by Mark Hamill,
Carrie Fisher, Harrison Ford, et al, release date May 21, 1980

3   "Tigger," n.d. Winnie the Pooh, Disney, Accessed April 20, 2019, https://
    winniethepooh.disney.com/tigger

4   Author's comment: On-island and off-island are island slang phrases for being on
    or away from the island. They are similar to being in or out of town.

5   Joe Dispenza, 2018, "In Order to Change Your Life, YOU NEED TO LEARN
    THIS FIRST! (Eye Opening Speech)," YouTube, Be Inspired, June 20, 2018,
    https://www.youtube.com/watch?v=wvWUpHv4AXs&vl=en
    Full interview by Tom Bilyeu of Impact Theory at www.youtube.com/
    watch?v=wvWUpHv4AXs&vl=e

6   Petsinger, Kerry. 2019. "Feeling Stuck in Life? How to Never Get Stuck Again."
    Lifehack. Lifehack. November 26, 2019. https://www.lifehack.org/630925/
    feeling-stuck-is-not-fun-this-is-how-i-never-feel-stuck-in-life-again

7   "Joyce Carol Oates Quotes (Author of We Were the Mulvaneys)," n.d. Goodreads,
    Goodreads. Accessed December 8, 2019, https://www.goodreads.com/author/
    quotes/3524.Joyce_Carol_Oates

8   "Joyce Carol Oates Quotes (Author of We Were the Mulvaneys)," n.d. Goodreads,
    Goodreads. Accessed December 8, 2019, https://www.goodreads.com/author/
    quotes/3524.Joyce_Carol_Oates

Endnotes - Chapter 16

1   Bernice Buresh, and Sioban Nelson, From Silence to Voice: What Nurses Know
    and Must Communicate to the Public (3rd Edition), Cordell Unity Press, 2013

2   Tim Mc Clure, "Videos & Events," Tim McClure, Accessed July 06, 2019

3   House, Oriah "Mountain Dreamer" from THE INVITATION (c) 1999.
    Published by HarperONE, San Francisco. All rights reserved.
    Presented with permission of the author. www.oriah.org

4   Marianne Williamson, "A Quote from A Return to Love,"
    Goodreads, Accessed July 06, 2019, https://www.goodreads.com/
    quotes/928-our-deepest-fear-is-not-that-we-are-inadequate-our

5   Emoto, Masaru, and David A. Thayne. 2011. Secret Life of Water. New York:
    Atria Books

6   Ariza-Montes, Antonio, et al. "Workplace Bullying among Healthcare Workers."
    MDPI, Multidisciplinary Digital Publishing Institute, 24 July 2013, www.mdpi.
    com/1660-4601/10/8/3121/htm

7   Vipula Gandhi, 2019, "Want to Improve Productivity? Hire Better Managers,"
    Gallup.com.,Gallup, April 20, 2019, https://www.gallup.com/workplace/238103/
    improve-productivity-hire-better-managers.aspx

8   "Self Realization is the Highest Healing" 2017, YouTube, The Chopra Wellness
    Center. August 22, 2017. https://www.youtube.com/watch?v=NHh1s4-OaCE
    Author's comment: I highly recommend watching the full video and others
    associated with it. The specific information cited is found at the 21:23 to 22:28
    time interval of the video.

9   Ironside, M.; Seifert, R. Tackling bullying in the workplace: The collective
    dimension. In Bullying and Emotional Abuse in the Workplace: International
    Perspectives in Research and Practice; Einarsen, H., Hoel, H., Cooper, C., Eds.;
    Routledge: New York, NY, USA, 2003; pp. 383–398. [Google Scholar]

10 Daniel Zwerdling, "Hospital To Nurses: Your Injuries Are Not Our Problem," NPR, NPR, February 18, 2015, https://www.npr.org/2015/02/18/385786650/injured-nurses-case-is-a-symptom-of-industry-problems

11 Tom Rath and Jim Hester, 2010, "The Economic of Wellbeing," Rep. The Economics of Wellbeing, Gallop Press
Authors are co-authors of, *Wellbeing: The Five Essential Elements*, published 2010

12 Carol Vallone Mitchell, "A Cautionary Tale for Tall Poppies and Women Leaders," The Huffington Post, TheHuffingtonPost.com, 7 Dec. 2017, www.huffingtonpost.com/carol-vallone-mitchell/a-cautionary-tale-for-tal_b_11266084.htm on 7 Jan. 2020 found at https://www.huffpost.com/entry/a-cautionary-tale-for-tal_b_11266084

13 ibid

14 A Quote by R. Buckminster Fuller," n.d. Goodreads, Goodreads, Accessed May 11, 2018

15 The History of Wartime Nurses: Duquense University," Duquesne University School of Nursing, Accessed July 06, 2019, https://onlinenursing.duq.edu/history-wartime-nurses/

16 Collins, MSN, RN, Rhonda. "Bring Nurses Back to the Bedside." For the Record, Great Valley Publishing Company, Inc, 1 Sept. 2015, www.fortherecordmag.com/archives/0915p10.shtml Vol. 27 No. 9 P. 10

17 "Institute of Medicine to Become National Academy of Medicine." National Academy of Science, Engineering and Medicine, Office of News and Public Information, 28 Apr. 2015

18 Committee on the RWJF Initiative on the Future of Nursing, "The Future of Nursing: Leading Change, Advancing Health" - NACNS," Accessed May 6, 2018, http://www.nacns.org/wp-content/uploads/2016/11/5-IOM-Report.pdf

19 ibid

20 ibid

21 ibid

22 "Chapter Two: The Quest For True Belonging." Braving the Wilderness: the Quest for True Belonging and the Courage to Stand Alone, by Brown Brené, Thorndike Press, a Part of Gale, a Cengage Company, 2018

23 "The Future of Nursing 2020-2030." National Academy of Medicine, 30 July 2020, nam.edu/publications/the-future-of-nursing-2020-2030/

24 Brené Brown, Dare to Lead: Brave Work, Tough Conversations, Whole Hearts, Random House, 2018

25 "Dare to Lead Quotes by Brené Brown," n.d. Goodreads, Goodreads, Accessed June 11, 2019, https://www.goodreads.com/work/quotes/62183586-dare-to-lead-brave-work-tough-conversations-whole-hearts

26 Ali Binazir, 2011, "Why You Are A Miracle." HuffPost, HuffPost, August 16, 2011, https://www.huffpost.com/entry/probability-being-born_b_877853

27 ibid

28 Marianne Williamson, "Our Deepest Fear" (poem), A Return to Love: Reflections on the Principles of A Course in Miracles, HarperPerennial, 2012, ©1992

29   "The Hand That Rocks the Cradle (Poem) by William Ross Wallace." Wikipedia, Wikimedia Foundation, 28 May 2018, en.wikipedia.org/wiki/The_Hand_That_ Rocks_the_Cradle_(poem)
"The Hand That Rocks the Cradle Is the Hand That Rules the World" is a poem by William Ross Wallace that praises motherhood as the preeminent force for change in the world. The poem was first in 1865 under the title "What Rules the World". The refrain of the poem is a commonly quoted phrase. Read the complete poem at http://www.theotherpages.org/poems/wallace1.html

30   ibid

31   Williamson, "Our Deepest Fear".
Author's note: Paraphrased and adapted from Marianne Williamson's poem, words in brackets modified or added to emphasize point of view.

32   Frederick Buechner, n.d. "A Quote from Wishful Thinking: A Theological ABC," Goodreads, Goodreads, Accessed May 17, 2018, https://www.goodreads.com/ quotes/140448-the-place-god-calls-you-to-is-the-place-where

Endnotes - Chapter 17

1   "Neville Goddard Quotes (Author of Power of Awareness)." n.d. Goodreads. Goodreads. Accessed December 7, 2019. https://www.goodreads.com/author/ quotes/53919.Neville_Goddard

2   "Hero's Journey," 2020, Wikipedia, Wikimedia Foundation, March 29, 2020, https://en.wikipedia.org/wiki/Hero's_journey: Conceptualized by Joseph Campbell, an American mythological researcher, who discovered several common stages that almost every hero-quest goes through regardless of culture. Here is a fun video summary https://youtu.be/GNPcefZKmZ0

3   Murdock, Maureen. 2020. The Heroines Journey. Boston, MA: Shambhala.

4   "A Quote by Guillaume Apollinaire ," n.d. Goodreads, Goodreads, Accessed May 7, 2018, https://www.goodreads.com/author/quotes/66522.Guillaume_ Apollinaire
Authors note: I have attempted to attribute this accurately via credible resources. There are several variations in verbiage, punctuation and some deliberation of its author. This source and version are on framed artwork I have owned since 1996, I cannot account whether the artist may have taken some creative liberty with the words even though it includes the credit to Guillaume Apollinaire 1870-1918. This version supports the spirit of my intended use; whether you think you are ready or not–stress and all–Life calls, organizes and pushes.
Another variation- General Discussion :: The Poetry Archives @eMule. com, Accessed July 10, 2019, http://www.emule.com/2poetry/phorum/read. php?4,34313 Come to the edge. We might fall. Come to the edge. It's too high! COME TO THE EDGE! And they came, and he pushed, and they flew. Christopher Logue (1926-)

5   "A Quote by Guillaume Apollinaire ," n.d. Goodreads, Goodreads, Accessed May 7, 2018, https://www.goodreads.com/author/quotes/66522.Guillaume_ Apollinaire
Authors note: I have attempted to attribute this accurately via credible resources. There are several variations in verbiage, punctuation and some deliberation of its author. This source and version are on framed artwork I have owned since 1996, I cannot account whether the artist may have taken some creative liberty with the words even though it includes the credit to Guillaume Apollinaire 1870-1918.

This version supports the spirit of my intended use; whether you think you are ready or not–stress and all–Life calls, organizes and pushes.
Another variation- General Discussion :: The Poetry Archives @eMule. com, Accessed July 10, 2019, http://www.emule.com/2poetry/phorum/read. php?4,34313 Come to the edge. We might fall. Come to the edge. It's too high! COME TO THE EDGE! And they came, and he pushed, and they flew. Christopher Logue (1926-)

6   "A Quote by Albert Einstein," n.d. Goodreads, Goodreads, Accessed May 7, 2018, https://www.goodreads.com/quotes/987-there-are-only-two-ways-to-live-your-life-one
     Authors note: I have attempted to attribute this accurately via credible resources. There are however several variations in verbiage, punctuation and apparently some deliberation around its author.

7   "A Course in Miracles – Chapter 1: The Meaning of Miracles – I. Principles of Miracles," n.d. A Course in Miracles (Book), Foundation for Inner Peace, Living Church Ministries, Inc. (blog). Accessed April 11, 2019, https://acourseinmiraclesnow.com/course-miracles-principles-miracles/

8   Scott, Elizabeth, "Science-Backed Links Between Health And Happiness," Verywell Mind, Verywell Mind, March 17, 2020, https://www.verywellmind.com/the-link-between-happiness-and-health-3144619

9   "World Happiness Report 2020," World Happiness Report, Sustainable Development Solutions Network, March 20, 2020, https://worldhappiness. report/

10   Matt Matt O'Brien, "New Report Says a Quarter of All U.S. Jobs Will Be Disrupted by Artificial Intelligence," Inc.com. January 24, 2019, Accessed January 26, 2019, https://www.inc.com/associated-press/new-report-says-quarter-of-us-jobs-will-be-replaced-by-ai.html

11   015, "How Disease-Based, Doctor-Centered Medicine Is Failing Us: Rx: The Quiet Revolution: WTTW," Rx: The Quiet Revolution, David Grubin, April 16, 2015

12   "Gospel of Thomas Saying 48." n.d. Gospel of Thomas Saying 48 - GospelThomas.com. Accessed December 7, 2019. http://www. earlychristianwritings.com/thomas/gospelthomas48.html

ACKNOWLEDGMENTS & GRATITUDE

My hug, Steve, thank you for listening, for years, to my dream of writing a book and supporting me as I walked the winding road toward it and then through the process. I love you.

My dearest friends and *Soul Sistahs*, women who are intuitive, dynamic, intelligent and inspirational with whom I am deeply blessed to walk through life: Susan, Cindy and Diane, also amazing nurses in a spectrum of innovative capacities. Carol, who is also my creativity and accountability friend. And Marcy who is a loving mother with perception, inner strength and resilience that is amazing to me. Thanks to each of you for the many adventures, lively phone conversations, for asking challenging questions, picking me up, cheering me on and for your love.

Angela Lauria of the Authors Way as my initial manuscript writing mentor along with the editors and staff at the Author Castle. Thank you for guiding me through those amazing first steps of drafting this book and helping me attain my amethyst author wings.

Julie Beyers, my editor, Thank you for your stick-to-it-ness, discernment, honesty, encouragement and for seeing it my way sometimes. I could not have polished my manuscript into this amazing book without you.

David Loofbourrow, for skillfully nurturing the dance of creativity between the members of our book production team, and for being able to bring into manifestation what we imagined using your expertise in cover, book design and typesetting… and humor. You, Julie and I have become kindred spirits in life, purpose, relationship, health and creativity.

Sharon Darrow, Vice President and past president of Northern California Publishers and Authors (NCPA) for sharing her experience and knowledge.

Norma Thornton, NCPA Communications Director & Newsletter Editor, for her enthusiastic encouragement and the other members of NCPA for their inspiration through authorship and insights.

Rev. Dr. Betsy Schwarzentraub, secretary and past president of Gold Country Writers (GCW), for her insightful chapter review and feedback on the spiritual foundations of the AH-SUCCESS process. Congratulations to her for publishing her third book, *Growing Generous Souls: Becoming Grace-Filled Stewards* with her fourth about to arrive.

Thank you to the many other generous and gifted members of GCW for their inspiration and encouragement.

Stephan Rechtschaffen, MD, president and co-founder of the Omega Institute in Rhinebeck, New York, for the privilege to work with and learn from him and the faculty of his holistic studies institute. Most deeply for sharing his guidance and inspiring me to write a book contributing my knowledge for the good of the whole – an achievement he had each of his faculty accomplish.

I have included the words, comments, insights, proposals, and research of many people and some organizations in this book, which by doing so, does not imply agreement or association between parties, but rather to honor how each contributed to my learning, inspiration, and growth.

Thank you authors, researchers, songwriters, poets, healers, visionaries, and my colleagues, patients, family and friends from whom I have learned, been inspired and loved – and you, reader.

ABOUT THE AUTHOR

Barbara Young is the author of *The Heart that Rocks Health Care*, the Easy as A-B-C Technique and the AH SUCCESS Process of transforming stress into success. For over thirty-five years, she has assisted people with self-awareness, regulation and care for stress recovery and well-being. Her 'Conscious Living Education' has been the foundation of her practice since the early 1990s. She 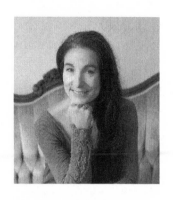 co-developed and taught an Integrative Healing Arts program used by nurses and patients for self-regulation of human responses to stress at a Northern California community hospital in 2016-17.

Among her nursing specialty certifications, she holds a board certification as a Holistic Nurse and Vascular Access Specialist and a BS in Nursing with a minor in Psychology. She is an ordained minister, a masters and doctoral candidate at the University of Sedona, a mind body skills educator, Certified Integrative Healing Arts Practitioner, Reiki Master, massage therapist and HeartMath® practitioner and mentor/coach with experience and training in many modalities.

She has found that, "Nurses are the conduit of care that allows any profession, hospital, business, organization or technology to touch people." Barbara has thrived beyond serious stress related auto-immune symptoms with self-regulation, using food as medicine and professional guidance from practitioners of Functional and Naturopathic Medicine as partners in her health care.

She divides her time between Northern California and the Caribbean and is available for education, mentoring and speaking. You can contact her or find other written works at www.BYoungBooks.com.

The first edition of this book, *The Heart that Rocks Health Care: Nurses, Move from Stress to Success, Empowerment and Influence*, earned Amazon's number one best-seller recognition as a new release in 2018

Made in the USA
Columbia, SC
13 October 2021

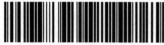

46908672R00238